A PRACTICAL MANUAL OF HYSTEROSCOPY AND ENDOMETRIAL ABLATION TECHNIQUES

A CLINICAL COOKBOOK

A PRACTICAL MANUAL OF HYSTEROSCOPY AND ENDOMETRIAL ABLATION TECHNIQUES

A CLINICAL COOKBOOK

RESAD P. PASIC, M.D., Ph.D.

Associate Professor of Obstetrics, Gynecology & Women's Health
Assistant Director, Section of Operative Gynecologic Endoscopy
University of Louisville School of Medicine
Louisville, Kentucky

RONALD L. LEVINE, M.D.

Professor of Obstetrics, Gynecology & Women's Health
Director, Section of Operative Gynecologic Endoscopy
University of Louisville School of Medicine
Louisville, Kentucky

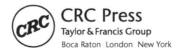

CRC Press
Taylor & Francis Group
Boca Raton London New York

CRC Press is an imprint of the
Taylor & Francis Group, an **informa** business

A TAYLOR & FRANCIS BOOK

CRC Press
Taylor & Francis Group
6000 Broken Sound Parkway NW, Suite 300
Boca Raton, FL 33487-2742

First issued in paperback 2019

ISBN-13: 978-1-84214-224-0 (hbk)
ISBN-13: 978-0-367-39422-6 (pbk)

British Library Cataloguing in Publication Data

Data available on application

Library of Congress Cataloging-in-Publication Data

Data available on application

Composition by Parthenon Publishing

Visit the Taylor & Francis Web site at
http://www.taylorandfrancis.com

and the CRC Press Web site at
http://www.crcpress.com

We dedicate this book to the memory of Dr. Jay Cooper and other modern day pioneers of hysteroscopy, several of whom have contributed chapters to this publication.

It is because of their persistence, vision, expertise and the application of scientific principles in their research, that our patients benefit from the advantages of hysteroscopy.

CONTRIBUTING AUTHORS

LINDA D. BRADLEY, M.D.

Director of Hysteroscopic Services
Department of Obstetrics and Gynecology
Cleveland Clinic Foundation
Cleveland, Ohio

MARLIES Y. BONGERS, M.D., Ph.D.

Maxima Medical Center
The Netherlands

PHILIP G. BROOKS, M.D.

Clinical Professor
Geffen School of Medicine at UCLA
Attending Physician – Cedars-Sinai Medical Center
Los Angeles, California

GINGER N. CATHEY, M.D.

Fellow of Operative Gynecologic Endoscopy
Department of Obstetrics, Gynecology & Women's
  Health
University of Louisville School of Medicine
Louisville, Kentucky

LAURA CLARK, M.D.

Associate Professor of Anesthesiology
University of Louisville School of Medicine
Louisville, Kentucky

JAY M. COOPER, M.D.

Women's Health Research
University of Arizona School of Medicine
Department of Obstetrics and Gynecology
Phoenix, Arizona

KEVIN G. COOPER, M.Sc, M.D., M.R.C.O.G.

Consultant Gynaecologist
Aberdeen Royal Infirmary
Aberdeen, Scotland, UK

ANDREW L. DE FAZIO, M.D.

Fellow, Atlanta Center for Special Pelvic Surgery,
  Gynecology, Endocrinology & Endometriosis
Atlanta, Georgia

HERVÉ FERNANDEZ, M.D.

Professor of Gynecology, Obstetrics and
  Reproduction
University Paris
Hospital Antione Beclere
Cedex, France

MILTON H. GOLDRATH, M.D.

Associate Professor
Department of Obstetrics and Gynecology
Wayne State University School of Medicine
Women's Health Care Physicians
West Bloomfield, Michigan

RICHARD J. GIMPELSON, M.D., P.C.

Assistant Clinical Professor
Department of Obstetrics and Gynecology
St. Louis University School of Medicine
Chesterfield, Missouri

KEITH B. ISAACSON, M.D.

Director of Minimally Invasive Surgery and
  Infertility
Newton Wellesley Hospital
Newton, Massachusetts

SARI KIVES, M.D.

Assistant Professor of Obstetrics and Gynecology
University of Toronto
Toronto, Ontario
Canada

RONALD L. LEVINE, M.D.

Professor of Obstetrics, Gynecology & Women's
 Health
University of Louisville School of Medicine
Director, Section of Operative Gynecologic
 Endoscopy
Louisville, Kentucky

BEVERLY R. LOVE, M.D.

Chairman of Surgery at Crosby Memorial Hospital
Assistant Medical Director at The Women's Clinic
Picayune, Mississippi

DANIELA MARCONI, M.D., Ph.D

Department of Obstetrics and Gynecology
S. Giuseppe Hospital
Rome, Italy

ROOSEVELT MCCORVEY, M.D.

Medical Director – Women's Wellness Center
Montgomery, Alabama

MALCOLM G. MUNRO, M.D.

Professor of Obstetrics and Gynecology
David Geffen School of Medicine at UCLA
Attending Physician – Kaiser Foundation Hospitals
Los Angeles Medical Center
Los Angeles, California

CEANA NEZHAT, M.D.

Director, Atlanta Center for Special Pelvic Surgery,
 Gynecology, Endocrinology & Endometriosis
Atlanta, Georgia

RESAD P. PASIC, M.D., Ph.D.

Associate Professor of Obstetrics, Gynecology &
 Women's Health
Assistant Director, Section of Operative Gynecologic
 Endoscopy
University of Louisville School of Medicine
Louisville, Kentucky

ALESSIO PIREDDA, M.D.

Department of Obstetrics and Gynecology
S. Giuseppe Hospital
Rome, Italy

JOSEPH S. SANFILIPPO, M.D., M.B.A.

Professor of Obstetrics, Gynecology & Reproductive
 Sciences
The University of Pittsburgh School of Medicine
Vice Chairman of Reproductive Services
Magee-Women's Hospital
Pittsburgh, Pennsylvania

EUGENE V. SKALNYI, M.D.

Vice President of Medical Affairs
Novacept, Inc.
Palo Alto, California

JONATHON SOLNIK, M.D.

Assistant Clinical Professor
Division of General Obstetrics and Gynecology
University of California at Irving
Irving, California

RAFAEL F. VALLE, M.D.

Professor of Obstetrics and Gynecology
Northwestern University Medical School
Chicago, Illinois

GEORGE A. VILOS, M.D.

Professor of Obstetrics and Gynecology
The University of Western Ontario
St. Joseph's Health Care
London, Ontario
Canada

ERRICO ZUPI, M.D.

"Tor Vergata" University of Rome
Department of Obstetrics and Gynecology
Fatebenefratelli Hospital
Rome, Italy

PREFACE

In 2002, we published a book on laparoscopy entitled *A Practical Manual of Laparoscopy: A Clinical Cookbook.* At first, the name of the book was criticized greatly; however, its merits became apparent and subsequently it was widely accepted as an easy to read and understandable text – the title became a mark of edification.

We were then encouraged to edit a book on hysteroscopy along the same vein that could be used by physicians in training, but would also serve as a handy reference for practicing physicians. This book continues in the style of the laparoscopy text, using the outstanding digital images created by Branko Modrakovic based on photos and drawings of the individual chapter authors. Each chapter has been written by experts in hysteroscopy who are renowned for not only their knowledge, but also their ability to teach.

Hysteroscopy, although known since 1869 and used since 1925, has gained general acceptance by gynecologists relatively slowly. It wasn't until 1970 when 32% Dextran was used to distend the uterine cavity, that gynecologists slowly began to utilize hysteroscopy, not only for diagnosis, but also for operative procedures.

Many other techniques have subsequently been developed since 1981, when Goldrath and colleagues published data on the use of hysteroscopy to ablate the endometrium with a laser. This opened the gates for the everyday gynecologist to offer alternatives to hysterectomy in the treatment of severe meno-metrorrhagia.

The hysteroscope also permits the outpatient treatment of many other pathologies including sub-mucosal leiomyomas, endometrial polyps, uterine synechia and uterine septa. Recently, hysteroscopic sterilization techniques have been developed and widely accepted as office based procedures.

This book has chapters that address all of the present hysteroscopic therapies and will provide an in depth discussion of the current knowledge of hysteroscopy and global ablation techniques.

The reader will note that many topics may appear to be repetitious as the individual chapter authors were allowed to express their views of procedures. There are also some differences in opinion as to techniques. We believe that allowing the freedom to disagree, even in the same book, is in itself, an educational benefit and will expose the reader to a more balanced view of current knowledge. We, the editors, also may not be in complete agreement with some of the views expressed by the chapter authors; however our role is to educate not censor.

RESAD P. PASIC, M.D., Ph.D.
RONALD L. LEVINE, M.D.

FOREWORD

Not so many years ago hysteroscopy was known as a procedure in search of an indication. Much has changed since then, and now hysteroscopy has a broad range of diagnostic and therapeutic indications, which is only fitting, considering that early attempts to peer into the uterus predated early laparoscopy. It has always seemed strange, at least to me, that gynecologists persist in performing grasping procedures, curettage, biopsy, and deliver energy into the organ of our chief interest without the aid of visualization. Would you allow an orthopedic surgeon to do the same in your knee without an arthroscope? Ardent hysteroscopists will tell you that the ability to make an instant diagnosis in an office, often with direct treatment has changed management of abnormal uterine bleeding. Office-based hysteroscopic uterine canalization as a tool to open corneal blockage in cases of infertility spawned the technology to accomplish the opposite; office transuterine sterilization is no longer a horizon topic, but an approved, effective method to permanently occlude the Fallopian tubes. Hysteroscopic uterine septum incision, described herein by one of the world's masters, Dr Valle, has rendered the hysterotomy route obsolete.

Flush on the heels of their widely acclaimed book on laparoscopy, Drs Pasic and Levine have applied the same logic and template to produce a similar work on hysteroscopy, which happily includes a chapter on saline infusion sonography as a related diagnostic technique. Described as a "cook-book" approach, the text serves as an excellent primer for the neophyte as well as for those with experience who are interested in expanding their repertory of operative interventions. Cook books come in various formats. Some are lavishly illustrated, but quickly become beautiful coffee table ornaments, never to be put to actual use in the kitchen. Others furnish the ingredients, quantities, time in the oven, but are devoid of helpful hints. The best practical cook book tells you what to use and in what amount, sequentially how to do it, pitfalls to avoid, and has illustrations that make the point. As such, a hysteroscopic Julia Child would laud this work. The chapters are informative and concise. The illustrations, actual photos or line drawings, deliver the message. The reader quickly grasps what to do, and just as importantly, what not to do. New

methods of endometrial ablation are clearly detailed, with appropriate pros and cons.

Over 2.5 million visits are made annually to gynecologists in the United States because of menorrhagia. Instructive texts such as this open diagnostic and therapeutic doors outside traditional hospital settings with great savings of time, money and a tremendous reduction of patient anxiety. Combined endometrial ablation and sterilization, which can be accomplished simultaneously in a matter of minutes, allow us to vastly improve the quality of life for our patients.

STEPHEN L. CORSON, M.D.

ACKNOWLEDGEMENTS

As editors, we were totally dependent upon the individual chapter authors. The list of authors reads like a who's who in hysteroscopy and we are extremely grateful for their diligence and outstanding contributions.

We are also extremely grateful for the financial support and for the graphic material supplied by the following members of the instrument manufacturing community:

ACMI Corporation

American Medical Systems

Boston Scientific

Conceptus, Incorporated

Cook Ob/Gyn

Gynecare, A Division of Ethicon, Inc.

Karl Storz Endoscopy

Microsulis Americas Inc.

Novacept

Olympus

Richard Wolfe Medical Instruments Corporation

We also must thank the Department of Obstetrics, Gynecology and Women's Health for their continuing encouragement and support.

This book, as well as our other contributions to the medical literature, would not be possible with out the hard work and long hours spent by our executive secretary Ms. Laura Lukat-Coffman and our editorial assistant Ms. Leta Weedman. We cannot thank them enough.

CONTENTS

SALINE INFUSION SONOGRAPHY

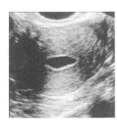

Linda D. Bradley, M.D.

The introduction of intracervical fluid during TVUS (Transvaginal Uterine Sonography) constitutes one of the most significant advances in ultrasonography during this past decade. Instillation of saline during ultrasound (SIS) enhances and augments the image of the endometrial cavity, as well as provides valuable information about the uterus and adnexa in patients with abnormal bleeding. Given the disparity between endometrial biopsy results and TVUS evaluation, pathologic reports including: "insufficient tissue," "atrophic endometrium," or "scant tissue" on biopsies are no longer sufficient to rule out pathology. SIS provides an exquisite view of the endomyometrial complex that cannot be obtained with TVUS alone. SIS differentiates between focal and global processes and improves the overall sensitivity for detecting abnormalities of the endometrium.

Saline infusion sonography overcomes the limitations of traditional TVUS for evaluating menstrual and postmenopausal bleeding disorders. It offers the advantages of distending the uterine walls to create a three-dimensional view of the uterus, and provides a more concentrated visualization of the endometrium and myometrium. This information helps to determine whether endometrial biopsy is needed, select the type of surgical procedure, ascertain the hysteroscopic expertise required to remove the lesions, and judge the resectability of lesions.

Saline infusion sonography is a procedure whereby saline is infused into the endometrial cavity during TVUS to enhance the endometrial view. Although many terms have been used to describe this technique (e.g., echohysteroscopy, hydrosonography, sonohysterography, sonohysterosalpingography, sonoendovaginal ultrasonography) the acronym SIS, saline infusion sonography, was coined by Widrich, Bradley and Collins in 1996, and more clearly defines the technique employed.

In comparison to hysteroscopy, SIS more reliably predicts depth of myometrial involvement of uterine fibroids and their size. For a successful surgical outcome, it is important to identify preoperatively the size, number, location, and depth of intramural extension. Fibroid size and location affect resectability, the number of surgical procedures necessary for complete resection, the duration of surgery, and the potential complications from fluid overload. SIS classification was developed for uterine fibroids, based on the purpose of planning surgery, determining resectability of lesions, and to standardize the comparison of surgical outcomes.

CLINICAL ROLE OF SALINE INFUSION SONOGRAPHY IN THE EVALUATION OF MENSTRUAL DISORDERS

COMMON INDICATIONS FOR PERFORMING SIS:

- EVALUATION OF MENSTRUAL DISORDERS IN THE PREMENOPAUSAL OR POSTMENOPAUSAL PATIENT.

- EVALUATION OF THE ENDOMETRIUM WHEN IT IS POORLY VISUALIZED, THICKENED, IRREGULAR, OR NOT IMAGED WELL BY CONVENTIONAL TVUS, MRI OR CAT SCAN STUDIES.

- EVALUATION OF A BIZARRE, IRREGULAR, OR INHOMOGENEOUS ENDOMETRIUM IN WOMEN ON TAMOXIFEN.

- EVALUATION OF PATIENTS WITH RECURRENT PREGNANCY LOSS OR INFERTILITY.

- POST SURGICAL EVALUATION OF THE ENDOMETRIUM.

- THE NEED TO DIFFERENTIATE BETWEEN SESSILE AND PEDUNCULATED MASSES OF THE ENDOMETRIUM.

- TO EVALUATE THE SURGICAL FEASIBILITY OF HYSTEROSCOPIC MYOMECTOMY.

- TO ASCERTAIN THE CLASSIFICATION OF UTERINE FIBROIDS (SIZE, NUMBER, LOCATION).

- CLARIFY FINDINGS WITH HYSTEROSALPINGOGRAM (HSG).

- EVALUATION OF RECURRENT PREGNANCY LOSS.

- PRESURGICAL EVALUATION OF INTRACAVITARY FIBROIDS, TO DETERMINE THE DEPTH OF MYOMETRIAL INVOLVEMENT AND OPERATIVE HYSTEROSCOPIC RESECTABILITY.

- POST SURGICAL EVALUATION OF THE ENDOMETRIUM.

- TO DETERMINE ENDOMETRIAL CHANGES DUE TO TAMOXIFEN.

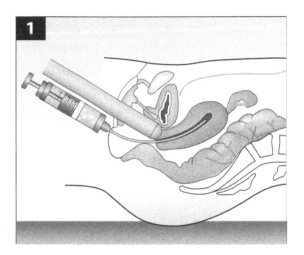

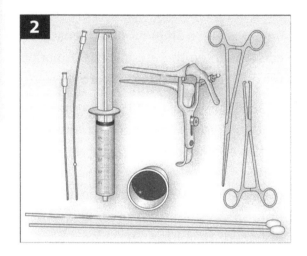

SIS TECHNIQUE

Although SIS can be performed transvaginally or transabdominally, most physicians use the transvaginal approach (Figure 1). No anesthesia or analgesia is required. Most patients are very comfortable. This procedure is best scheduled when the patient is not bleeding. Reproductive aged women ideally should be scheduled during the early proliferative phase – preferably 4–10 days after menses has ended. The risk of interrupting a viable intrauterine pregnancy is lowest at this time. Additionally, fewer false positive results, and fewer artifacts caused by shearing of the endometrial cavity will occur. Visualization of endometrial polyps and fibroids is enhanced during the early proliferative phase.

PREPARATION

The required instruments are shown in Figure 2. Antibiotics are not routinely given except for patients who have symptoms or signs of pelvic infection, prior history of pelvic inflammatory disease, mitral valve prolapse, cardiac valves, or artificial hips. Patients may elect to use nonsteroidal anti-inflammatory drugs (NSAIDs) one to two hours before the procedure. Thus, SIS requires minimal preparation and no anesthesia. Women with cervical stenosis may benefit from placement of laminaria tents or misoprostol (orally 100 mcg 8 to 12 hours before the procedure or vaginally 200 mcg to 400 mcg 6 to 8 hours before the procedure). Uterine sounding may sufficiently disrupt synechiae. Cervical traction with a single-toothed tenaculum can straighten the uterine axis if marked retroversion is present (Figure 3).

Voiding before SIS is important. Bladder distention is not required. In fact, it can alter the position of an anteverted uterus to retroverted, making evaluation with a transvaginal probe onerous. After informed consent is obtained, a bimanual examination is performed with the patient in the dorsal lithotomy position. An absorbent towel placed under the patient will minimize fluid accumulation.

Conventional TVUS is performed using a transvaginal probe covered with a condom and gel. Visualization of the cervix is aided by placing an open-sided speculum in the vagina to facilitate introduction of the intrauterine catheter and permit easy removal of that same speculum without displacing the catheter.

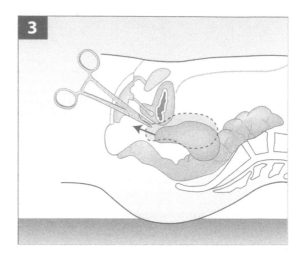

The cervix is cleansed with an antiseptic solution, such as Betadine or Hibiclens. The intrauterine catheter then is inserted with the assistance of a ring forceps or uterine forceps.

The catheter should be placed to barely touch the fundus. Several flexible intrauterine catheters that provide easy access to the endometrium are currently available. I prefer the 25-cm long, 5.6 F Soules which is a 1.8 mm (Cook Ob/Gyn, Indianapolis, IN) intrauterine insemination catheter. It is inexpensive and easy to use and place within the uterus. Its long length allows extension through the introitus, which permits easy attachment of a sterile syringe. For conditions such as incompetent cervix, Asherman's syndrome, or patulous cervix, a balloon-type catheter is useful to optimize uterine distention and minimize fluid loss (Figure 4).

Before the catheter is inserted, it is flushed with sterile saline to decrease artifacts caused by bubbles. A straight catheter should be introduced with sterile uterine packing forceps until the fundus is reached. If distention is inadequate, it may be helpful to pull the catheter back. When cervical stenosis is encountered, a tenaculum or uterine sound can be used to assist in placing the catheter.

After the open-sided speculum is removed, the Soules catheter will protrude from the vagina, allowing easy attachment of a 60 mL plastic syringe containing sterile saline. Air bubbles should be evacuated from the syringe also, to prevent artifacts.

SIS is a dynamic procedure, and images are best seen in real time. Excellent images and adequate distension usually are obtained with minimal fluid instillation (5–30 mL). Ideally, 5 to 10 mL/min are infused. If the uterus cannot be distended, placing a balloon-tipped catheter and infusing the saline more slowly may help. Air bubbles may accumulate but rapidly disappear as the injection continues. More fluid can be safely used if the patient is bleeding or has blood clots, or if there is poor visualization.

It is essential to employ a systematic technique for viewing the uterus and to watch the video monitor as the scan is performed. As the endometrial cavity unfolds on the screen, it is important to view the uterus as a three-dimensional structure that must continually be recreated as scanning continues. This three-dimensional image is achieved by scan-

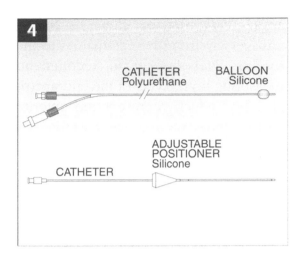

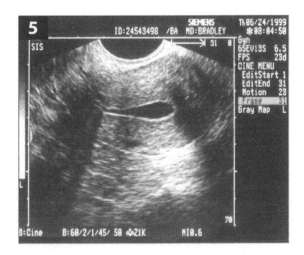

ning from cornua to cornua in the long axis (sagittal plane) (Figure 5) and then turning the probe 90° and scanning from the endocervix to the fundus in the transverse plane (Figure 6). The sagittal view permits visualization of the uterine cavity and measurement of the endometrial echo. The adnexa are visualized in the semi coronal plane. The cervix and cul-de-sac are viewed as the transducer is withdrawn. Uterine symmetry and myometrial or intracavitary lesions are appreciated best by slowly scanning transversely from the external os to the fundus. Fleischer et al recommend measuring both layers of the endometrial echo (which represent the anterior and posterior uterine wall basal layers) in the sagittal view to obtain the most accurate measurement of the endometrium. The hypoechoic subendometrial halo should not be included because it represents the vascular layer of myometrium. Both TVUS and SIS can be performed in 10–15 minutes in most patients.

FINDINGS

ENDOMETRIAL POLYPS

Endometrial polyps occur frequently in the reproductive and menopausal years. They more commonly occur in women on tamoxifen. Polyps are usually single, falsely widen the endometrial echo when imaged with TVUS alone, do not disrupt the endomyometrial complex and appear homogeneous with microcystic changes (Figure 7). Sometimes cystic spaces within an abnormally thickened endometrium tend to be predictive of polyps.

INTRAUTERINE FIBROIDS

Fibroids are difficult to locate with conventional TVUS because they transmit sound poorly, attenuate the beam, and have ill-defined borders. Fibroids may obscure measurements of the

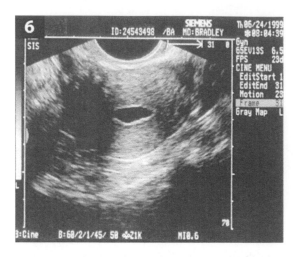

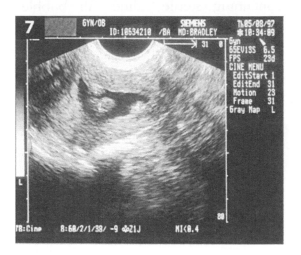

endometrium by creating an irregular endomyometrial interface. They may have varied appearance, including cystic, calcific, hypoechoic, echogenic, isoechoic, and mixed echogenic patterns. Degenerating fibroids often appear cystic. Location of fibroids is improved with SIS. The endometrium adjacent to the fibroid appears echogenic. Additionally, location, size, and degree of intramural extension can be classified with SIS.

The following classification of intra-cavitary uterine fibroids based on SIS was developed for the purpose of planning surgery. Notice that this classification differs from the hysteroscopic classification described in Chapter 12. SIS Class 1 fibroids are intracavitary and do not involve the myometrium. The base or stalk is visible with SIS (Figure 8).

SIS Class 2 fibroids have a submucosal component that involves less than 50% of the myometrium (Figure 9). The size of the fibroid does not influence the classification system, solely its location. The difference between class 2 and class 3 fibroids is in the extent of the intramural involvement. The extent of the intramural involvement is measured by ultrasound.

SIS Class 3 fibroids have an intramural component greater than 50%. They can be transmural and located anywhere from the submucosa to the serosa. These fibroids often appear as a bulge or indentation into the submucosa when viewed hysteroscopically (Figure 10).

For a successful surgical outcome, it is important to identify preoperatively the size, number, location, and depth of intramural extension of uterine fibroids. SIS offers certain advantages to hysteroscopy in evaluation of intrauterine fibroids. The exact size and depth of intramural involvement can be assessed and measured by ultrasound. The thickness of the myometrium over the myoma can also be assessed and

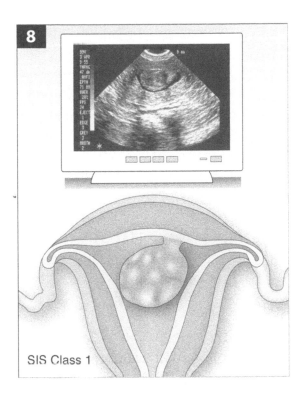

SIS Class 1

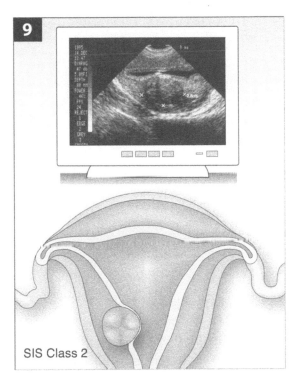

SIS Class 2

measured. Fibroid size and location are associated with complete resectability, the number of surgical procedures necessary for complete resection, the duration of surgery, and the potential complications from fluid overload. Proper preoperative evaluation of the size, location and number of fibroids may help the surgeon to decide if a laparoscopic approach is more suitable than hysteroscopic resection.

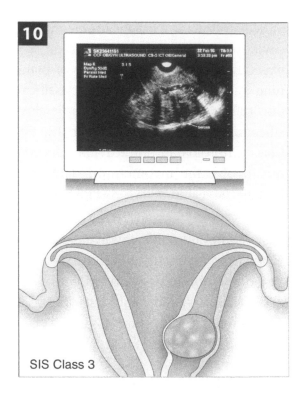

SIS Class 3

CLASSIFICATION OF INTRACAVITARY UTERINE FIBROIDS BASED ON SIS:

- SIS CLASS 1 FIBROIDS ARE INTRACAVITARY AND DO NOT INVOLVE THE MYOMETRIUM. THE BASE OR STALK IS VISIBLE WITH SIS.

- SIS CLASS 2 FIBROIDS HAVE A SUBMUCOSAL COMPONENT THAT INVOLVES LESS THAN 50% OF THE MYOMETRIUM.

- SIS CLASS 3 FIBROIDS HAVE AN INTRAMURAL COMPONENT GREATER THAN 50%. THEY CAN BE TRANSMURAL AND LOCATED ANYWHERE FROM THE SUBMUCOSA TO THE SEROSA.

ENDOMETRIAL ATROPHY

An atrophic endometrium is typically observed in menopausal women and in those with prolonged Depo-Lupron, Depo-Provera, and continuous oral contraceptive use. In postmenopausal women, atrophic endometrium produces a pencil-thin endometrial echo less than 5 mm thick. Atrophic endometrium can easily be identified by SIS as shown in Figure 11.

ENDOMETRIAL HYPERPLASIA

Endometrial hyperplasia cannot be definitively diagnosed with SIS, however endometrial thickness, echogenicity, and appearance may suggest the need for endometrial biopsy for confirmation or hysteroscopy. Endometrial hyperplasia can only be documented by histologic analysis. Hyperplasia may be global, multifocal, focal, or occur within a polyp. Hyperplasia may produce a uniformly hyperechoic and thickened endometrium (Figure 12).

ENDOMETRIAL CANCER

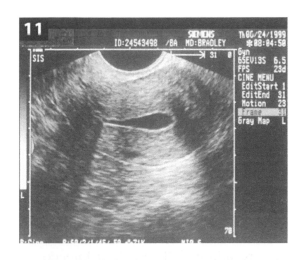

Endometrial cancer requires a histologic analysis, however it can be suspected by the increased endometrial thickness by TVUS or characteristic appearances obtained with SIS (Figure 13). The endometrial echo has a myriad of appearances in patients with endometrial cancer, including an irregularly thickened, ill-defined endometrium; a heterogeneous pattern; and mixed echogenicity with variable hypoechoic texture. The endomyometrial junction may be intact or irregular. Endometrial cancer is difficult to distinguish from hyperplasia unless the endometrial thickness is increased or associated with a disruption of the endomyometrial interface.

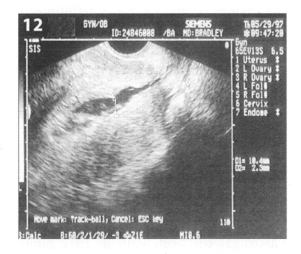

INTRAUTERINE ADHESIONS

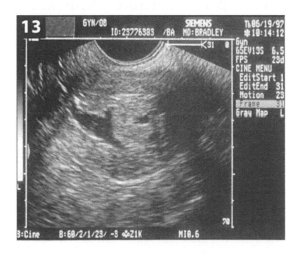

Shalev et al, demonstrated better appreciation of intrauterine adhesions during midcycle compared to menses. Intrauterine adhesions appeared as hyperechoic, irregular, linear echoes, with cordlike features and endometrial foci that could be differentiated from polyps by their irregular shape and more precise location. Adhesions interrupt the continuity of the endometrial layer (Figure 14). In patients with Asherman's syndrome, the adhesions appear as thin, bridging bands that may distort the endometrium. In addition, the uterus may be difficult to distend.

POTENTIAL PROBLEMS AND TROUBLESHOOTING OPTIONS

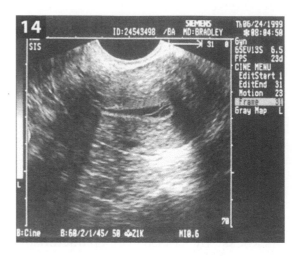

The procedural risks associated with SIS are minimal. The risk of infection is less than 1%. Practitioners should follow the same protocols for administering antibiotics as they do with hystero-salpingogram or other invasive endometrial procedures. A bimanual examination and visual inspection of the cervix should be performed before any instrumentation. If bacterial vaginosis, trichomonas, or other sexually transmitted diseases (STDs) are suspected, the procedure should be abandoned.

Cervical manipulation can produce a vasovagal reaction. Patients may rarely experience bradycardia, dizziness, or severe pain; therefore, resuscitative equipment should be readily available.

There are no published reports of uterine perforation with SIS. The procedure causes minimal pain, but non-steroidal anti-inflammatory drugs (NSAIDs) can be administered 1 to 2 hours preprocedure if desired, although this does not appear to significantly decrease the already low pain scores.

The possibility of transmitting metastatic endometrial cancer through the fallopian tubes during SIS is purely speculative. The small amounts of fluid used and the low infusion intrauterine pressure will minimize risk to the patient. Historical data on patients with endometrial cancer evaluated by hysterosalpingography found no evidence or worse than normal outcomes.

False positive results with SIS may be caused by blood, debris, clots, thickened endometrial folds, secretory endometrium, detached fragments of endometrium, or endometrium that may be sheared during placement of the catheter. When SIS is performed in the presence of active uterine bleeding, endometrial clots may sometimes be mistaken for polyps, fibroids, or hyperplasia. Because false positives may lead to unnecessary surgical intervention, SIS should be performed when these are least likely. Appointment secretaries and nursing staff are critical in the scheduling process. For premenopausal women, that means scheduling SIS within 1 to 7 days completion of the menstrual cycle. In postmenopausal women, the patient should be scanned when she is not bleeding, if possible. If she is taking sequential hormone replacement therapy (HRT), SIS is best performed after progesterone withdrawal.

POSTPROCEDURE INSTRUCTIONS

Saline infusion sonography is associated with few complications. Most patients are able to leave the office within 15 minutes of the procedure and return to work and activities. Since narcotics are not generally used, patients may drive alone and do not require an escort. Patients are instructed to refrain from vaginal intercourse for 24 hours. In the event of increased temperature, foul-smelling discharge, or persistent pelvic pain, patients should contact their physician. Prompt re-evaluation is imperative.

SUGGESTED READING:

Widrich T, Bradley L, Mitchinson AR, Collins R. Comparison of saline infusion sonography with office hysteroscopy for the evaluation of the endometrium.
Am J Obstet Gynecol 1996;74:1327-1334

Cincinelli E, Romano F, Anastasio P, et al. Transabdominal sonohysterography, transvaginal sonography, and hysteroscopy in the evaluation of submucous myomas.
Obstet Gynecol 1995;85:42-47

Emanuel MH, Verdel MJ, Wamsteker K. A prospective comparison of transvaginal ultrasonography and diagnostic hysteroscopy in the evaluation of patients with abnormal uterine bleeding: Clinical implications. Am J Obstet Gynecol 1995;172:547-552

Bradley LD, Falcone T, Magen A. Radiographic imaging techniques for the diagnosis of abnormal uterine bleeding. Obstet Gynecol Clinics North America 2000;27(2):245-276

Preutthipan S, Herabutya Y. Vaginal misoprostol for cervical priming before operative hysteroscopy: A randomized controlled trial. Obstet Gynecol 2000;96:890-894

Dessole S, Farina M, Capobianco G, Nardelli GB, Ambrosini G, Meloni GB. Determining the best catheter for sonohysterography. Fert Steril 2001;76(3):60:605-609

Fleischer AC, Kalemeris GC, Machin J, et al. Sonographic depiction of normal and abnormal endometrium with histopathologic correlation. J Ultrasound Med 1986;5:445-452

Hulka CA, Hall IDA, McCarthy K, Simeone JF. Endometrial polyps, hyperplasia, and carcinoma in postmenopausal women: differentiation with endovaginal sonography. Radiology 1994;191:755-758

Gaucherand P, Piacenza JM, Salle B, Rudigoz RC. Sonohysterography of the uterine cavity; preliminary investigations. J Clin Ultrasound 1995;23(6):339-348

Weigel M, Friese K, Strittmatter HJ. Measuring the thickness-Is that all we have to do for sonographic assessment of endometrium in postmenopausal women? Ultrasound Obstet Gynecol 1995;6:97-102

Shalev J, Meizner I, Bar-Hava I, Dicker D, Mashiach R, Ben-Rafael Z. Predictive value of transvaginal sonography performed before routine diagnostic hysteroscopy for evaluation of infertility. Fertil Steril 2000;73(2) 412-417

Cullinan JA, Fleischer AC, Kepple DM, Arnold AL. Sonohysterography; a technique for endometrial evaluation. Radiographics 1995;15(3):501-514

Mihm LM, Quick VA, Brumfield JA, Connors AF, Finnerty JJ. The accuracy of endometrial biopsy and saline sonohysterography in the determination of the cause of abnormal uterine bleeding. Am J Obstet Gynecol 2002;186:858-60

HYSTEROSCOPIC INSTRUMENTS

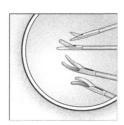

Ronald L. Levine, M.D.

Many instruments are available for the hysteroscopist. Instruments which may be used for a particular procedure, such as global therapy instruments, will be described in each chapter (See chapters 14–18). In this chapter we will only describe instruments for general use:

Hysteroscopes and Sheaths;

Fluid Management Systems;

Accessory Instruments;

Resectoscopic Instruments;

Ancillary Equipment;

Light source;

Energy source.

1. HYSTEROSCOPES AND SHEATHS

Hysteroscopes may be divided into two general subcategories: Rigid and Flexible.

RIGID HYSTEROSCOPES

This type of hysteroscope is the one most commonly used for operative hysteroscopy but in its simplest form it may be used only for diagnostic hysteroscopy. The rigid hysteroscope system is comprised of a telescope that is not used by itself and therefore requires an outer sheath for instilling the distension media. The conventional hysteroscopic sheath attaches to a matched 3–4 mm telescope. Simple diagnostic sheaths have only an inflow port to permit the distension media to be infused (Figure 1).

The sheaths may be complex with inflow and outflow valves (Figure 2). The conventional single-flow hysteroscopic sheath is outfitted with two oppositely positioned stopcocks that are open to the same channel. Distension medium and operative instruments share a common route (Figure 2). Newer diagnostic sheaths accommodate liquid media by virtue of independent inflow and outflow tracts for so-called continuous flow. This allows for continuous flushing and rinsing of the uterine cavity. Sheaths that have continuous flow capabilities may also have ancillary working channels that usually span from about 1 mm (3 Fr) to about 2.3 mm

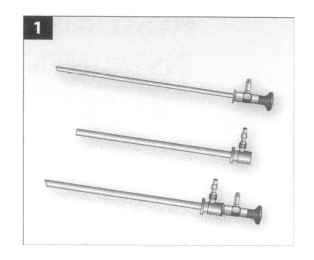

THE RIGID HYSTEROSCOPES

- OUTER DIMENSION RANGES 2–4 mm & LENGTH OF 35 cm

- ROD LENS SYSTEM

- COLD ILLUMINATION

- MAGNIFICATION INVERSELY RELATED TO DISTANCE

- BRINGING THE TELESCOPE CLOSER OR FARTHER MAGNIFIES OR REDUCES THE IMAGE.

- PANORAMIC VIEW OF 60–90°

- FIELDS OF VIEW: CENTERED LENS = 0°, OFFSET 12°, 25°, OR 30°

- ANGLE OF VIEW OPPOSITE THE LIGHT POST

- OUTER DIAMETER OF DIAGNOSTIC SHEATH 3–5 mm

- OUTER DIAMETER OF OPERATIVE SHEATH 7–8 mm

(7 Fr) to allow the passage of operating instruments. Semirigid operative hysteroscopic instruments are preferable for operative hysteroscopic surgery. Classic configurations include scissors, biopsy forceps, and tissue graspers. The stopcocks are fitted with small rubber gaskets to prevent the fluid from coming out. The sheath itself will be from 3 to 8 mm outer diameter (O.D.) depending upon the system.

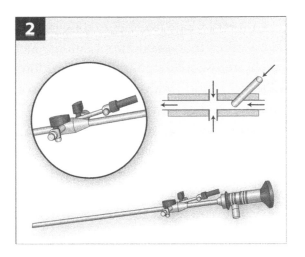

In an operating hysteroscope system, the outer sheath may be 7–8 mm O.D. A bridge connects the sheath to the telescope and permits insertion of 7 Fr caliber instruments. Some systems have an obturator with a blunt end inside the sheath so that the sheath can be passed without the scope inside, in a similar manner as a dilator is passed through the cervix. The obturator is then removed and the scope itself is placed within the sheath (Figure 3).

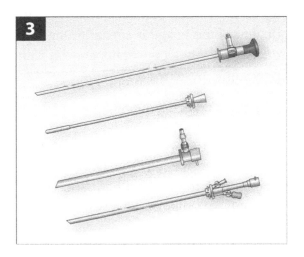

Rigid hysteroscopes usually come in a variety of sizes and in a variety of viewing capabilities, ranging from 0 degree to 30° fore-oblique angle. The view through the scope is in the opposite direction of the light post, i.e. if one is viewing through a 12° scope, you would be seeing 12° away from the light post (Figure 4). Most modern hysteroscopes contain a rod lens system rather than the old "bead" lens, permitting a brighter and clearer image. If a liquid distension medium is used, the depth of field will be about 2–3 cm.

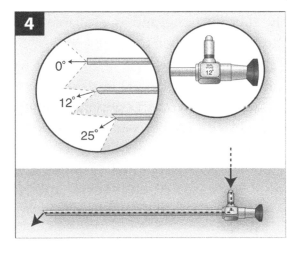

A 3 mm scope may be used by itself or with other therapeutic applications such as hysteroscopic sterilization procedures (Essure®) and with some endometrial ablation techniques (HTA™).

There are also semi-rigid micro diagnostic continuous flow hysteroscopes that when used with a sheath, have only 1.8 mm to 3 mm diameter and 12° angle of view. The VERSASCOPE is a flexible pixel telescope with an outer diameter of 1.8 mm and length of 28 cm providing 0° field of view. Illumination is provided by a standard fiber bundle system and the quality of the image is similar to that produced by the conventional rod lens panoramic hysteroscope.

CONTACT HYSTEROSCOPES

These are rigid instruments and are not very popular in the US. They do not require media or a light source and are only for diagnostic purposes. The instrument collects room light in a cylinder near the eyepiece. The light is then transmitted through a glass rod system. The instrument is approximately 200 mm long and is available in 6 and 8 mm diameters (Figure 5).

The magnification is small, only 1.6X and the view is limited to tissue that is close to the lens. An optional magnifying device may be used to provide an additional 2X magnification; however panoramic views are not possible. This is a very simple instrument and as noted above is only useful for diagnostic purposes.

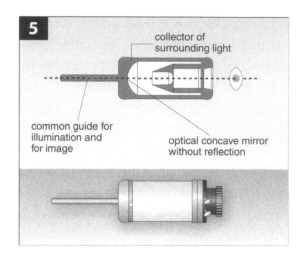

FLEXIBLE HYSTEROSCOPES

Flexible hysteroscopes are fiberoptic scopes that are primarily used for diagnostics; however, some of the larger diameter scopes can be used for some operative procedures. The operative channel is approximately 1.2 mm. Only flexible operative instruments can be used and they are rather fragile due to their small size and have only limited use.

The newer generation of fiberoptic scopes has an insertion diameter of about 3.1 mm (9 Fr) to 5.0 mm and a working length of about 240 mm. The scope may have a 90° to 100° field of view. The flexible scopes have a bar on the handle portion that permits the end of the scope to be angulated within the confines of the uterus to either bend up or down from 90° to 110° depending upon the manufacturer (Figure 6).

The light source for the flexible scope may be as small as a 175 to 250 watts halogen or xenon light as the new generation of flexible hysteroscopes have as many as 12,000 to 30,000 fibers per scope permitting good light within the endometrial cavity.

2. FLUID MANAGEMENT SYSTEMS

In hysteroscopy accurate control of pressure and distension media delivery is of utmost importance (See Chapter 3). Many surgeons use a simple system of hanging a fluid bag on an I.V. pole and using gravity to supply the pressure (Figure 7). The fluid bag should be positioned about 100 cm above the patient's uterus in order to provide adequate distention pressure. If the gravity is not good enough to provide adequate visualization of the uterine cavity, as in cases when operative procedures are performed, hysteroscopy pumps are utilized. The pump delivers constant chosen pressure for adequate distention of the uterine cavity (Figures 8). The pumps are accompanied with specialized tubing that connects to the inflow and outflow valves on the hysteroscope sheath.

They are combined irrigation and suction devices where intrauterine pressure can be set and regulated. They allow controlled and precise irrigation and distention of the uterine cavity by connecting to the inflow and the outflow valves of the hysteroscopy sheath. They are also accompanied with fluid collection bags that are taped to the

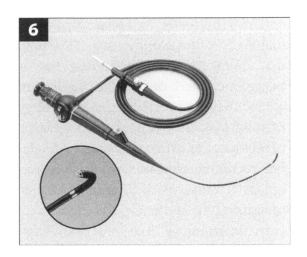

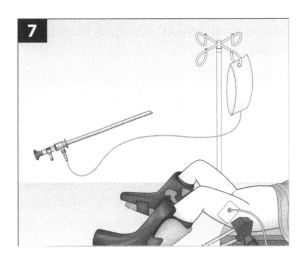

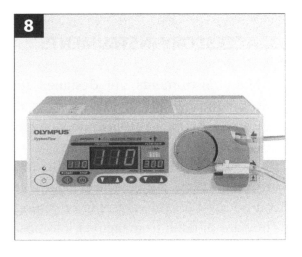

patient's buttocks to collect any fluid that escapes the uterine cavity. The fluid that drains into the collection bag is being suctioned out to the fluid management system for accurate assessment of fluid loss. The American Association of Gynecologic Laparoscopists (AAGL) has recommended mechanical monitoring as it removes the human factor in measuring fluid deficit and allows for early warning of excessive extravasations. Accurate and continuous monitoring of fluid inflow, outflow and deficit is the most effective way to decrease the risks associated with fluid overload.

There are several systems on the market that measure by weight the fluid bags and then weigh the recovered fluid to provide an accurate deficit reading (Figure 9). Fluid in bags may be 10% overfilled as allowed by law, thus creating the potential for a moderate error in estimating fluid absorption unless the bags are weighed. The intrauterine pressure can be set and is controlled automatically.

3. ACCESSORY INSTRUMENTS

Many instruments are designed for passing through the operating port of the hysteroscope. The instruments may be completely flexible, semi-rigid or rigid. As noted previously, flexible instruments are rather delicate but they can be used for fine grasping or cutting. They are difficult to maneuver into posi-

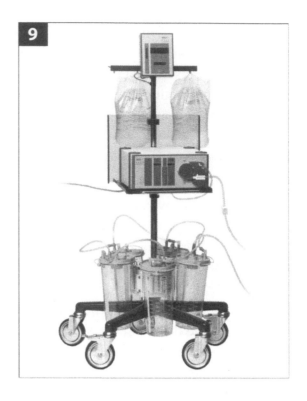

tion and therefore have limited use. Semi-rigid instruments include scissors, graspers and punch biopsy forceps. Although stronger than flexible instruments, they are still relatively fragile and only useful for removing small polyps or biopsies (Figure 10). These instruments are passed through the ancillary working channels with stopcocks that are fitted with small rubber gaskets to prevent the fluid from coming out of the hysteroscope sheath.

Rigid instruments are larger and therefore require a larger operative channel. Operative hysteroscopes with rigid instruments are called optical forceps. The optical forceps houses the scope and have scissor-like handles that operate the tip of the instrument (Figure 11). The rigid instruments are more sturdy and robust and may offer better assistance in removal of large polyps. They can be used when a strong mechanical advantage is required, such as the removal of an imbedded IUD. The instrument is already part of the hysteroscope sheath and the telescope is inserted along the instrument shaft to aid in the visualization of the instrument tip. The tip of the instrument can be in the form of scissors or forceps.

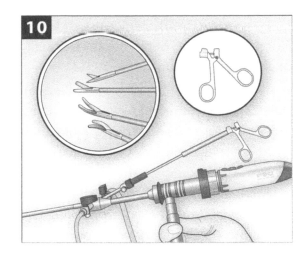

4. RESECTOSCOPIC INSTRUMENTS

The resectoscope has been used in bladder and prostate surgery by urologists for many years. Since 1990 it has been used in a slightly modified form by gynecologists to perform such operative procedures as excision of submucous myomas, endometrial polyps, division of uterine septa, and endometrial ablations (see Chapters 8, 12, 13).

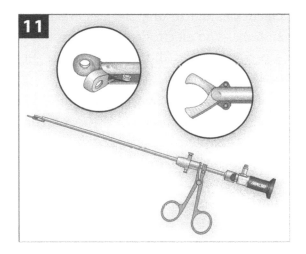

The resectoscope is comprised of five parts (Figure 12):

–The telescope with a 12° lens.

–A continuous flow outer sheath that has an inflow and an outflow stopcock. There are outflow holes located on the distal end of the sheath. The return flow empties between the two sheaths and through the outflow stopcock, which may in some cases be connected to suction, but more often is drained into a collecting bag. The resectoscopes require a larger continuous flow sheath (25–26 Fr).

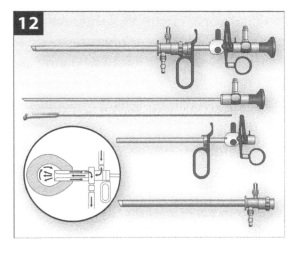

–An inner sheath, which is inside and connected to the outer sheath. It usually has an insulated tip.

–The working element is called an Iglesias-type element allowing one-handed operation. The working element is held with the fingers on the handgrip and the first digit of the thumb in the thumb ring. Pushing on the ring moves the electrode forward approximately 2 cm and the spring brings it back.

–Electrodes. There are a variety of electrodes for the resectoscope. Many electrodes utilize unipolar electrosurgical systems. The electrodes are connected to a power source (the electrosurgical generator) (Chapter 5).

The electrodes may be in the form of a wire loop that is utilized for resecting tissue (Chapters 12, 13). The wire loops may also come in different diameters ranging from .010 to .015 inch wire. The thinner the wire, the higher the power density and the faster it will cut and produce less coagulation; however, the thin wires will bend and break easily. There are three basic designs of monopolar resectoscopic electrodes. They are angulated up to 15° away from the optic to remain in the field of view during the operation. Cutting loops are primarily used to shave or remove submucous myomas.

Monopolar desiccation electrodes with ball or barrel configurations have substantially larger surface areas and are typically utilized to perform endometrial ablation and focal hemostasis.

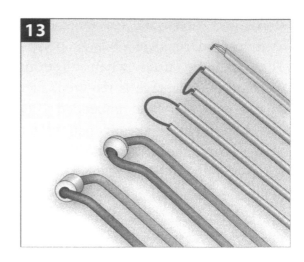

The roller ball, because of its smaller size, provides about 1 mm of surface contact as opposed to approximately 3 mm of contact area for the bar (Figure 13). The smaller size produces a higher power density and therefore a deeper burn but over a smaller area. Some electrodes have a different configuration.

There are some electrodes that are designed to produce a high power density that will vaporize the tissue rather than resect it. A barrel-shaped monopolar electrode that is periodically grooved can be effectively used to vaporize tissue. Each edge created by the grooves acts as a separate electrode, providing multiple doses of high density electrosurgical current to underlying tissue (Figure 14). This reduces the chips that result from resecting a myoma.

Some resectoscopes are made for the use of bipolar electrodes. The advantage of these systems is that they can be used with physiologic fluid distension media (normal saline) with the theoretical advantage of reducing the risk of hyponatremia (see Chapters 3, 20).

The VersaPoint™ bipolar system (Gynecare, Inc) consists of an active electrode, which is connected to a larger return electrode, all contained within a narrow sheath. The active electrode is available in several different configurations: a ball, a twizzle and a spring. Each is recommended for different usage (Figure 15).

The VersaPoint™ Resectoscopic System consists of a bipolar electrode and a dedicated resectoscope (Figure 16). This innovative instrumentation operates in normal saline solution distension medium for use in the treatment of benign uterine pathologies, such as polyps and submucosal fibroids.

The VersaPoint™ requires a specific bipolar generator that has three distinct modes of action: vaporization, desiccation and blend. The different settings on the generator create different size vapor pockets with decreasing voltage. For vaporization, the generator heats the saline around the active electrode, which creates an insulating vaporization pocket.

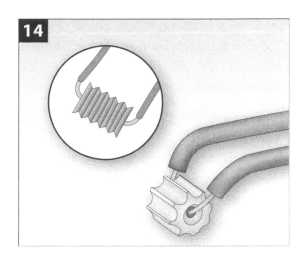

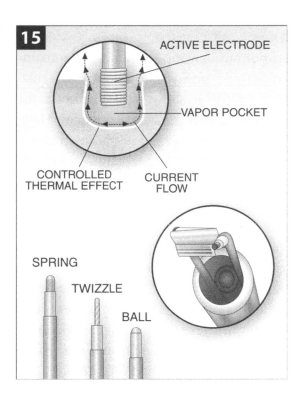

5. ANCILLARY EQUIPMENT

LIGHT SOURCE

The light is delivered to the hysteroscope usually via fiberoptic light cables, but some cables have a fluid medium to transmit the light. If not stored correctly, these fiberoptic cables may have broken fibers that can cut down greatly on the transmitted light. The origination of the light may be from either a tungsten halogen lamp of 175–250 W, a xenon lamp of

300 W or a halide lamp of 250 W (Figure 17). The halogen light is cheaper and is sufficient for the newer generation of hysteroscopes.

CAMERAS

The same cameras that are used for laparoscopic surgery can also be used for hysteroscopy. Modern video cameras all use solid-state microprocessor chips. The head attaches to the eyepiece of the hysteroscope and connects to the video controller by a cable (Figure 18). During hysteroscopy, it is extremely important that the camera head remains in a fixed position to avoid disorientation by the hysteroscopist. Because the uterine cavity is small, just a little change in the position of the camera can produce a rather large positional visual effect.

The quality of the image as seen on the monitor is related to the resolution of the camera and the monitor. The picture is only as good as the lowest resolution of either of the two elements. High definition endoscopic cameras and monitors have more than twice the number of scanning lines than the frame of conventional videos, therefore, producing a clearer image.

ENERGY SOURCES

LASERS: The use of lasers as an energy source in hysteroscopy has diminished over the last several years, although some centers still use a

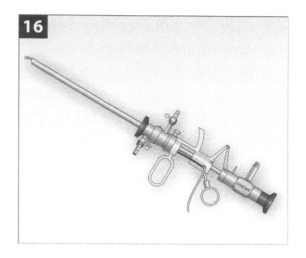

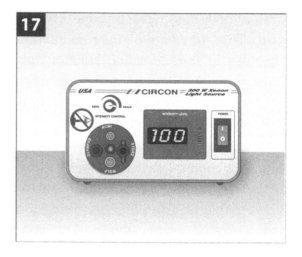

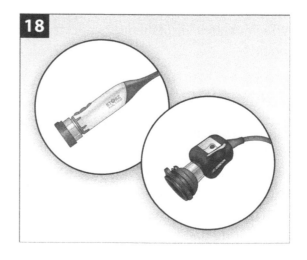

Nd:YAG (Neodynium. Ytrium, Aluminum, Garnet) laser with a wavelength of 1064 nm because it can transfer its energy through fluids to create good destruction of tissue. Delivery of this laser system requires the use of a quartz fiber approximately 0.6 mm in diameter. The skill needed to perform ablations with the laser requires a much steeper learning curve than the use of electrosurgical techniques and has a higher complication rate.

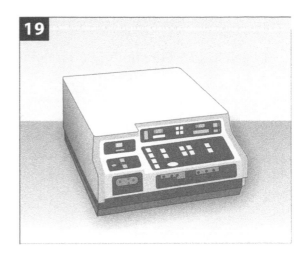

ELECTROSURGICAL UNITS

The electrosurgical generator, commonly called the "Bovie" is a high frequency or radio frequency alternating current generator. These generators have an output of over 100,000 Hz. Most generators have their output power displayed in Watts and have the ability to provide unipolar modulated and unmodulated current as well as bipolar circuits (Figure 19). The use of these generators is discussed in other chapters (See Chapter 5).

DISINFECTION AND HANDLING OF THE INSTRUMENTS

The hysteroscopic instruments should be handled with care due to the fragility of the telescopes and semi-rigid instruments. The instruments and telescopes should first be cleaned of debris and than disinfected using gas sterilization or soaked in 2% glutaraldehyde for at least 20 minutes. Fiberoptic cables should be disinfected along with the telescopes. Conventional hysteroscopic sheaths and rigid instruments should be autoclaved after being properly flushed and cleaned of blood products and debris. It is important always to follow manufacturer's guidelines for sterilization and disinfection.

PRINCIPLES OF DISINFECTION

- TELESCOPES
- DO NOT AUTOCLAVE
- GAS STERILIZATION
- SOAKING IN GLUTARALDEHYDE FOLLOWED BY RINSE
- AIR DRY BEFORE STORAGE

FIBER OPTIC CABLES

- GAS STERILIZATION
- SOAKING IN GLUTARALDEHYDE FOLLOWED WITH RINSE

SHEATHS AND RIGID INSTRUMENTS

- FLUSH AND CLEANSE
- AUTOCLAVE

RESECTOSCOPE

- FLUSH AND CLEANSE
- AUTOCLAVE

DISTENSION MEDIA IN HYSTEROSCOPY

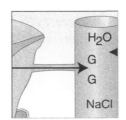

Philip G. Brooks, M.D.

Hysteroscopy provided precious little information concerning the causes of abnormal bleeding or reproductive problems until safe, effective distension was developed. What became evident was that, ideally, the distension medium had to allow the endometrial cavity to be opened, the view to be clarified (even in the face of blood), and little, if any, toxicity to the patient should the medium be absorbed into the vascular tree. In addition, the medium should be readily available at a minimal cost and be very compatible with the instruments used. Along with the dramatic advances in optics, light sources and documentation technologies, the advances in the development and utilization of different media have made hysteroscopy a standard tool for the evaluation and treatment of intrauterine pathologies.

CHOICE OF DISTENSION MEDIUM DEPENDS UPON:

- CLINICAL SETTING
- DIAGNOSTIC
- OPERATIVE
- ELECTROSURGERY
- MONOPOLAR VS BIPOLAR

GASEOUS MEDIUM: CARBON DIOXIDE

- HIGH VISCOSITY LIQUIDS: HIGH MOLECULAR WEIGHT DEXTRAN-70
- LOW VISCOSITY LIQUIDS: LOW MOLECULAR WEIGHT DEXTRAN
- GLUCOSE
- ELECTROLYTE-FREE SOLUTIONS: GLYCINE, SORBITOL, MANNITOL
- ELECTROLYTE-RICH SOLUTIONS: SALINE, LACTATED RINGER'S SOLUTION

TYPES OF MEDIA AVAILABLE

Contemporary hysteroscopy uses the following media for the distension of the uterus, each with its own special characteristics that make that medium useful for specific indications, and each with differing risks that limit its use:

IDEAL DISTENSION MEDIA

- ISOTONIC
- NON HEMOLYTIC
- NON TOXIC
- NON ALLERGIC
- RAPIDLY CLEARED
- AMPLE VISUALIZATION

CARBON DIOXIDE

Carbon dioxide is the only gaseous medium thought appropriate to use for uterine distension because it does not support combustion and has a wide margin of safety if absorbed into the blood stream at the low flow rates used in hysteroscopy. It is inexpensive, readily available in tanks and cartridges and has a refractive index the same as air, making the view exceedingly clear in the absence of blood and excessive mucus, both of which make bubbles that obstruct or distort the view. Disadvantages include the resultant shoulder pain if too much CO_2 gets into the peritoneal cavity through patent oviducts and the need for expensive special hysteroscopic insufflators to deliver the gas at the correct flow rate and pressure (Figure 1). While CO_2 has been widely used for diagnostic purposes, it is almost never helpful for operative procedures.

DEXTRAN-70 (HYSKON™)

Dextran-70 is a viscous solution, often requiring warming to be used hysteroscopically, and is readily available in 100 mL bottles. Its refractive index of 1.39 makes it a little more opaque and yellowish than air or water, but its density makes it nonmiscible with blood and generally too thick to traverse the oviducts with ease. Because it is electrolyte-free it can be used with electrosurgical procedures, and it was preferred for intrauterine laser surgery.

The disadvantages of using Dextran-70 have made it very undesirable. Numerous reports of allergic reactions, from hives to anaphylactic shock, and of fluid overload with pulmonary edema from vascular intravasation, have resulted in the demand for different and safe fluids. Additionally, when Dextran-70 dries, it can caramelize or harden, damaging surgical instruments if they are not rinsed with hot water immediately after the procedure. Although mechanical pumps have been designed for delivering the thick liquid, they are largely unavailable at present, and hand-delivered instillation, using a large bore syringe, is the usual method of injecting the solution into the uterus. Measurements of pressures delivered by

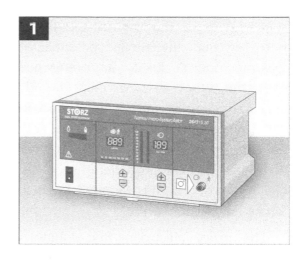

such hand-held instillation show that up to 450 mmHg can be achieved with this technique, adding further to the risks inherent with this distension method.

LOW VISCOSITY LIQUIDS

Low viscosity liquids require a system that allows continuous inflow and outflow because of their miscibility with blood and mucus. The fluid pressure can be regulated to obtain a maximum distension and facilitate better visualization of the uterine cavity. The system is also equipped with an outflow fluid collection bag that collects all the fluid coming out of the hysteroscope. By comparing the amount of fluid used and the amount of fluid collected in the system, the operator can determine the volume of fluid that has been absorbed in the patient's circulation. Some of the fluid monitoring systems are presented in Figures 2 and 3 (See Chapter 2).

Low-molecular weight Dextran, at 4% and 6% solutions, is available, but seldom is used. If a low viscosity liquid is to be used, the allergic potential of Dextran doesn't justify its preference over the other low viscosity liquids available. Glucose and dextrose historically have been used and can be very effective, but are rarely preferred over the more physiologic solutions or the electrolyte-free liquids required for hysteroscopic electrosurgery.

The major electrolyte-free solutions used for hysteroscopy are glycine, sorbitol and mannitol. Because they are electrolyte-free, they do not disperse electricity, thereby allowing electrical power to be delivered via the electrode to the intended tissue.

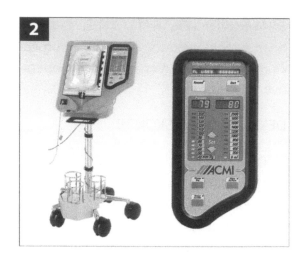

GLYCINE

Glycine was used for many years by urologists performing transurethral electrical resection of the prostate prior to the development of the resectoscope for gynecologic use. Glycine became the most frequently used distension medium for resectoscopic surgery because it was readily available in most institutions. It provides fairly good visibility, but like all nonviscous distension media it is miscible with blood and it requires a constant flow system. Glycine is a simple amino acid that is mixed with water as a 1.5% solution. Because it is both hypo-osmolor and hypotonic, if it intravasates into the vascular tree in significant amounts, it can produce profound hyponatremia and hyper-volemia,

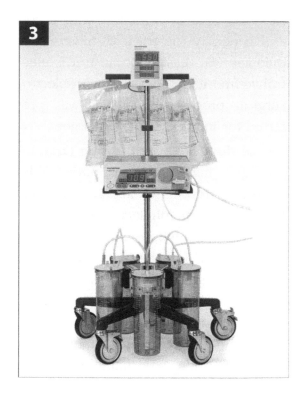

with pulmonary edema, edema of the brain, heart failure and death. A large intravascular bolus will eventually result in surplus of free water in the vascular space creating a hyponatremia (Figure 4). The glycine molecule has an intravascular half-life of 85 minutes, after which it is absorbed intracellularly (Figure 5). When glycine moves from the intravascular space into the cells it pulls the water from the vascular space to the interstitial space and intracellular space, causing brain edema (Figure 6). Cerebral edema may develop resulting in a compression of the brain against the skull. It is the only medium derived from amino acids; when it gets into the blood stream it breaks down to ammonia, possibly resulting in euphoria, transient blindness and coma.

SORBITOL AND MANNITOL

Sorbitol and mannitol are sugars, and are less hypo-osmolar and hypotonic, with mannitol being the safer of the two. Like glycine, they are non-electrolytic solutions and can be used for electrosurgery and they are miscible with blood and should therefore be used with constant-flow systems. Sorbitol is available in a 5% isotonic solution and is metabolized in the body to fructose and glucose.

Mannitol is also available in a 5% isotonic solution. The half-life of mannitol in plasma is 15 minutes. It is not metabolized in the body and it is excreted intact through the renal system resulting in additional osmotic diuresis. Mannitol acts rapidly as an osmotic diuretic theoretically reducing the risk of water overload. If significant intravasation occurs, the risk of hyponatremia still remains but the danger of hypervolemia is less.

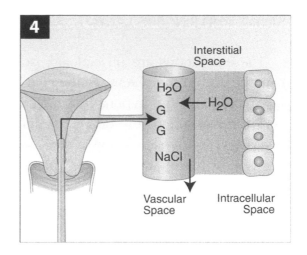

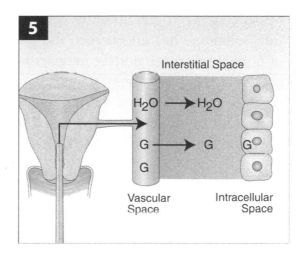

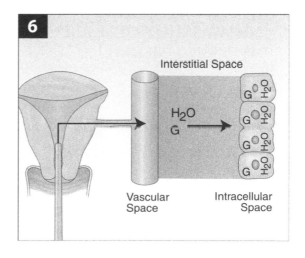

SALINE AND RINGER'S LACTATE

These solutions are physiologic, iso-osmolar and isotonic. As such they have less risk of creating hyponatremia. Until very recently, they were only used during diagnostic hysteroscopy or in conjunction with intrauterine laser procedures, as the presence of electrolytes precluded the use of these solutions during monopolar electrosurgical operations. The recent development of bipolar intrauterine surgery, explicitly designed to avoid the use of electrolyte-free solutions, has encouraged the use of normal saline solution for intrauterine surgery. Again, as these solutions are miscible with blood and mucus, continuous flow instrumentation is needed to keep the field in which to work clear.

FACTORS AFFECTING THE INTRAVASATION OF LIQUID DISTENSION MEDIA

- Intrauterine pressure
- Length of surgery
- Resection of large myoma
- Resection of large septum
- Partial perforation

PREVENTION OF COMPLICATIONS FROM DISTENSION MEDIA

Virtually nothing in medicine or surgery is entirely risk free! Most of the complications of operative hysteroscopy derived from the use of distension media can be prevented or minimized by understanding their causes and the techniques to prevent and manage them.

PREVENTION OF COMPLICATIONS

- Be familiar with the properties of the media that is used
- Monitor fluid balance
- Keep low intrauterine pressure (< 70 mmHg)
- Avoid closing the outflow valve
- Decrease the surgery time
- Avoid Trendelenburg position

Carbon dioxide, at flow rates used in hysteroscopy, is exceedingly safe. Insufflators, especially designed for use in hysteroscopy, being lower flow but higher pressure as compared to laparoscopy insufflators, must be used. Studies in both German shepherd dogs and in sheep revealed that, even if carbon dioxide is insufflated directly into the venous system at hysteroscopy flow rate and pressure, because of its high solubility in plasma, systemic changes barely occur even over a very long period of time. If bubbles occur during the use of CO_2 the flow rate should be decreased until the bubbles disappear, not increased with the intent of blowing the bubbles away, as is the natural tendency.

With the great availability of dual-channel, continuous flow instruments, there should be no significant need for the use of high-molecular weight Dextran-70. It is difficult to use because of its thickness and stickiness, and the potential for serious allergic reactions makes it very undesirable. Skin testing for allergy is possible but rarely performed for this use. The volume of Dextran-70 used and that retained by the body must constantly be monitored. Each 100 mL absorbed into the vascular system can expand the volume by 800 mL and, thus, can cause serious hyper-volemia (Figure 7). The manufacturer recommends extreme caution if more than 250 mL of Dextran-70 is required during a procedure.

Low viscosity liquids – glucose, saline, Ringer's lactate, glycine, sorbitol and mannitol – rarely cause allergic reactions, are more physiologic, and generally are safer to use for diagnostic or operative hysteroscopy. Because they are miscible with blood, they are

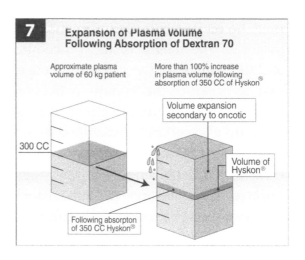

7 Expansion of Plasma Volume Following Absorption of Dextran 70

Approximate plasma volume of 60 kg patient

More than 100% increase in plasma volume following absorption of 350 CC of Hyskon®

300 CC

Volume expansion secondary to oncotic

Volume of Hyskon®

Following absorpton of 350 CC Hyskon®

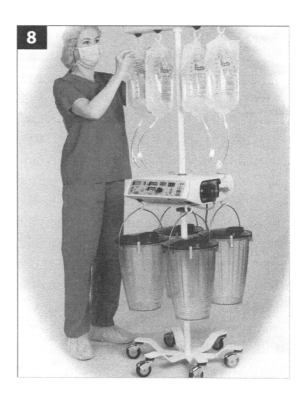

almost always used with continuous-flow circulating sheaths. However, whether the distension fluid contains electrolytes or not, the volume of liquid retained in the patient's blood stream must be minimized! Surgeons must be aware of the length of the procedure and the volume of the fluid used versus that retrieved in the outflow collection bottles. Because the three-liter bags of fluid are allowed to be overfilled by up to 10%, and because outflow collection canisters contain lines that are only approximate measures, it is mandatory to use one of the several types of mechanical fluid monitoring systems available (Figure 8 – See Chapter 2). This will allow almost constant awareness of the fluid deficit before it becomes a critical amount. The potential sources of fluid loss during hysteroscopy are shown in Figure 9. Published recommendations for allowable fluid deficits are between 1000 and 1500 mL for healthy women and 750 mL for those with compromised cardiovascular function. As stated above, the development of bipolar intrauterine electrosurgery using saline as the distension medium has reduced the risk of fluid overload by eliminating the hyponatremia. However, even excessive intravasation of saline solution has been reported to result in fluid overload, with congestive heart failure and/or pulmonary edema. Other factors contributing to excessive fluid absorption include: using excessive intrauterine pressure; working with reduced outflow due to closure of the outflow channel; and increased inflow into the venous system due to steep Trendelenburg position of the patient

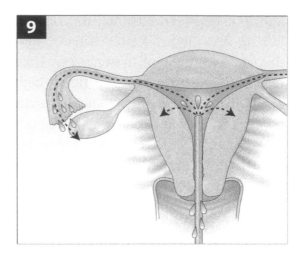

on the operating table, putting the heart below the level of the uterus, resulting in greater negative pressure in the veins.

TREATMENT OF SYMPTOMATIC HYPONATREMIA

- EARLY DETECTION AND RAPID INITIATION OF TREATMENT
- MONITORING OF ELECTROLYTES
- ADMINISTER LOOP DIURETIC SUCH AS FUROSEMIDE
- RESTRICT FLUID INTAKE
- SUPPLEMENTAL OXYGEN
- SERUM SODIUM <120 NMOL/L REQUIRES CRITICAL CARE SETTING
- SEEK TO CORRECT SERUM SODIUM GRADUALLY

CONCLUSION

Hysteroscopy, diagnostic or operative, requires the use of some distension medium in order to see clearly, work in the presence of blood, mucus or debris and allow mechanical surgery, laser surgery or electrosurgery to be performed. Each medium described here has unique properties and risks, all of which must be understood by the successful hysteroscopic surgeon to better perform the procedures with the greatest safety for his/her patient.

SUGGESTED READING:

Loffer F, Bradley L, Brill A, et al. Hysteroscopic fluid monitoring guidelines.
J Am Assoc Gynecol Laparosc 2000;7(1):167-198

Brooks P. Complications of operative hysteroscopy: How safe is it? Clinic Obstet
Gynecol 1992;35(2):256-261

Indman P, Brooks P, Cooper JM, et al. Complications of fluid overload from
resectoscopic surgery. J Am Assoc Gynecol Laparosc 1998;5:63-67

Witz CA, Silverberg KM, Burns WN et al. Complications associated with the absorption
of hysteroscopic fluid media. Fertil Steril 1993;60:745-56

CHOICE OF ANESTHESIA

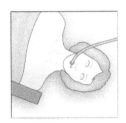

Laura Clark, M.D.

INTRODUCTION

Hysteroscopy presents unique anesthetic implications that have been learned through experience and with correlations from transurethral prostate procedures. Both the anesthesiologist and the gynecologist can initiate interventions that increase the safety and further the applications of this technique. This chapter will briefly address the anesthetic implications of hysteroscopy in general, but will focus on the unique aspects of hysteroscopy as different from other endoscopic procedures.

COOPERATIVE PLANNING
BETWEEN ANESTHESIOLOGIST AND SURGEON

Cooperation between the anesthesiologist and surgeon is vital, including their careful planning based on awareness of the physiologic and mechanical forces that lead to complications. Good communication and diligent attention to the monitoring of the patient leads to rapid detection of potential complications and successful outcomes with low complication rates.

SURGEON–ANESTHESIOLOGIST COLLABORATION

- THROUGH THE COURSE OF THE PROCEDURE

- MUTUAL AWARENESS OF CAUSES OF COMPLICATIONS

- GOOD COMMUNICATION PERIOPERATIVELY

- DILIGENCE IN MONITORING PATIENT

PREOPERATIVE ASSESSMENT

The surgeon and anesthesiologist should assess the patient's medical condition as soon as possible after the operation is scheduled so that the patient is referred appropriately and in a timely manner for optimization of the patient's medical condition prior to surgery. Oversight in this area is often a primary reason for cancellation of cases and is one of the easiest problems to correct.

Many studies have shown that a patient in optimal condition will experience less morbidity than those that come to surgery with inadequately treated pre-existing medical conditions. This is true even for the "healthy" female. The preoperative assessment of the patient is imperative for optimal outcome.

Prior to surgery, the patient's primary medical doctor should have recently evaluated medical conditions such as congestive heart failure, ischemic heart disease, diabetes, and hypertension. Often a referral to the primary care physician prior to surgery will expedite the patient's movement through the preoperative anesthesia evaluation and cause less delay in scheduling the patient for the operating room.

- THE SURGEON AND ANESTHESIOLOGIST SHOULD ASSESS THE PATIENT'S CONDITION AS SOON AS THE OPERATION IS PLANNED.

If the patient has significant medical problems, she should see the anesthesiologist prior to surgery for a preoperative anesthetic evaluation. At this time specific questions about anesthesia can be answered and specific instructions can be given to the patient regarding the immediate preoperative period. Most anesthesiologists like to instruct patients to avoid ACE inhibitors and diuretics the day of surgery. All other medications should be continued the day of surgery. Diabetics will need individualized instructions prior to surgery but usually will be instructed to hold insulin or hypoglycemic therapy the day of surgery.

NAUSEA AND VOMITING

At the preoperative interview the patient will be questioned for a prior history of postoperative nausea and vomiting. If other risk factors exist, such as motion sickness, smoking, or oral contraceptive use, multi-modal therapy may be indicated. These patients can be identified in the preoperative interview so that adequate treatment will be initiated the day of surgery. There are some studies suggesting the use of a scopolamine patch. Other studies have suggested the use of dexamethasone 4 mg. Another study indicated a lowered incidence of nausea and vomiting if 80% oxygen is used intraoperatively and supplemental oxygen is continued in the recovery room period. Nausea and vomiting are frequent reasons for postoperative admission. Every effort should be made to identify and appropriately treat these patients to avoid this costly and uncomfortable morbidity.

ANESTHETIC TECHNIQUE

The anesthetic technique will depend on the operation to be performed and the patient's condition. For diagnostic procedures, conscious sedation is often all that is necessary. The very anxious patient may require general anesthesia or regional anesthesia. General anesthe-sia with propofol may have a lowered incidence of postoperative nausea and vomiting when compared to inhalational agents. The use of a laryngeal mask airway should be reserved for selected cases performed with only a moderate Trendelenburg tilt in a non-obese patient. Tracheal intubation is the only way to truly protect the airway.

If the operation is extensive and/or the patient's medical condition warrants, invasive monitoring should be started preoperatively. Hypothermia can be significant if the fluids are not warmed, so a forced-air warming device may be employed. There are no studies that document a preferred method of anesthetic technique. One advantage of regional anesthesia is that the patient becomes his or her own best cerebral monitor. When unconscious with general anesthesia, the earliest signs and symptoms of fluid overload, dilutional hyponatremia, or gas embolism will not be evident. The use of a laryngeal mask airway would be an individualized decision based on the operation, the patient's medical history, body habitus and surgeon's technique. The use of laryngeal mask airway remains controversial.

- The choice of anesthesia depends upon the operation to be performed and the patient's condition.

TYPES OF ANESTHESIA

- LOCAL ANESTHESIA,
  WITH OR WITHOUT SEDATION
  (CONSCIOUS SEDATION)

- INFILTRATIVE BLOCK – SUBMUCOSAL
  OR PARACERVICAL

- REGIONAL – SPINAL OR EPIDURAL

- GENERAL

POSTOPERATIVE PAIN

Although hysteroscopy generally has little postoperative pain, many studies have concluded that a multi-factorial or multi-modal approach to postoperative pain yields the most satisfactory results. By approaching pain in this manner the total dose of opioids necessary is reduced. The lowered amount of opioids decreases their troublesome side effects. Opioids are undeniably a cause of nausea and vomiting, itching, excessive sedation and respiratory depression. A preoperative dose of a Cox-2 inhibitor has been shown to have an opioid-sparing effect and provide an adjunct to satisfy the total requirement for adequate pain control.

TRENDELENBURG POSITION

Deep Trendelenburg position is to be avoided during hysteroscopy. This position causes an initial drain of the elevated lower limbs' venous volume, resulting in increased preload. In the patient with a compromised cardiovascular system this increase could result in an overload to the heart. A Swan–Ganz catheter is not a reliable measure in the Trendelenburg position, and clinical impression should take precedence. It is best to avoid any Trendelenburg position to reduce the aspiration of air through opened vessels in the cervix and fundus by the negative pressure of the circulation. However, complications may occasionally arise as follows:

POTENTIAL PROBLEMS WITH TRENDELENBURG POSITION

- INCREASED PRELOAD

- SWAN–GANZ CATHETERS
  BECOMING UNRELIABLE

- HAMPERED OXYGENATION

- PULMONARY INADEQUACY

- UNPLANNED ONE-LUNG
  VENTILATION LEADING TO HYPOXIA
  AND PARTIAL LUNG COLLAPSE

PULMONARY EFFECTS OF TRENDELENBURG

The compression of viscera in this position can cause the diaphragm to move cephalad. This compression may increase the work of ventilation, resulting in increased airway pressure, decreased compliance, decreased vital capacity, and decreased functional residual capacity. Even healthy patients can see a 50% reduction in these values.

COMPLICATIONS FROM THE ANESTHESIOLOGIST POINT OF VIEW

Uterine perforation is probably the most common complication and is covered in the chapter on complications. It is important that both surgeons and anesthesiologists are familiar with the physiological impact of each medium and its potential complications, which can be severe to life threatening. Although fatal complications are quite rare, some degree of morbidity occurs in about 6% of patients.

GAS EMBOLISM AND CARBON DIOXIDE

Although gas embolism is more common with CO_2 insufflation during laparoscopy, it has been reported in hysteroscopy. Carbon dioxide in gaseous form is used as a medium only for diagnostic procedures, to avoid the high risk of gas embolism that would be present as many open vessels are created during surgical procedures. Carbon dioxide is used for the same reason that has made it a popular medium in laparoscopy – because it is noncombustible and highly soluble in blood. Nevertheless, one should not be com-

placent with its use in the diagnostic setting. There are reports of emboli with diagnostic use. In these reports, flushing air from the tubing with CO_2 dropped detectable emboli to near zero. It is still not known whether the emboli were due to CO_2 or air. A study comparing the use of CO_2 and normal saline suggested that endometrial malignant cells were introduced into the peritoneal cavity during hysteroscopy while using normal saline versus CO_2. The volume of gas necessary to produce symptoms is 25 mL/kg of CO_2 as opposed to 5 mL/kg of air.

Embolism generally occurs at the beginning of surgery. In a retrospective review of 3932 patients, the incidence was estimated at 0.03%, and a rate of 0.51% sub-clinical emboli. No emboli were reported in 1000 hysteroscopies when the tubing was flushed of air. To limit forced introduction of gas, a maximal distending pressure should be limited to less than 100 mmHg.

TREATMENT OF GAS EMBOLISM

Rapid detection and treatment are important to decrease morbidity from gas embolism. Often the first sign will be a rapid decrease in the expired CO_2 due to decreased cardiac output. This may or may not be coupled with a drop in oxygenation. Aspiration of gas, foamy blood from a central venous line, or air bubbles demonstrated on Transesophageal Echo (TEE) will provide definitive diagnosis. Other signs

Chapter 4

40 | CHOICE OF ANESTHESIA . . . .

of embolism include tachycardia, EKG sign of right heart strain, arrhythmias, and most ominously, hypotension and millwheel murmur. These last two can well indicate imminent cardiovascular collapse.

To help reverse the symptoms, place the patient in the head down and left lateral position to try to keep as much air as possible in the right atrium (Figure 1). Administer 100% oxygen with aspiration of as much gas as possible. Blood pressure should be supported while attempting to remove the air. Pretreatment with gonadotropin-releasing hormone (GnRH) agonists to reduce endometrial vascularity, avoidance of steep Trendelenburg, and careful deaeration of the equipment will further reduce the risk of gas embolism.

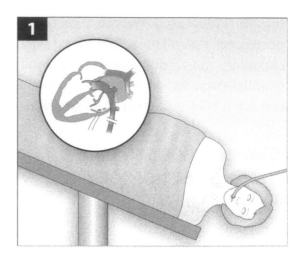

GAS EMBOLISM

- CHANGE PATIENT POSITION
- TRENDELENBURG POSITION
- GNRH PRETREATMENT
- 100% OXYGEN ADMINISTRATION
- DEAERATION OF EQUIPMENT

FACTORS UNIQUE TO HYSTEROSCOPY

As in any operation, the more involved the procedure, the greater the risk of complications. Hysteroscopy actually comprises a range of procedures from relatively benign diagnostic biopsy, requiring only light sedation, to involved surgical procedures under general anesthesia with complications potentially quite devastating to the patient. Recent advances in technique and knowledge have greatly lowered the incidence of complications, but there is always some risk. Indications for complexity of anesthesia and specific operations are discussed in other chapters of this book.

CONSCIOUS SEDATION

The service of an anesthesiologist is not necessarily required for diagnostic procedures. Usually, conscious sedation with local or topical anesthesia will suffice, but it places on the gynecologist both the burden of the procedure and the immediate welfare of the patient. For example, conscious sedation can rapidly progress to an undesirable level of sedation.

The gynecologist will need special preparation and vigilance in these cases knowing their limits as well as those of the patient. A full understanding of the patient's medical history is important to administer safe conscious sedation. They need to realize that some patients are not candidates for conscious sedation, even if the procedure that is prescribed for them could be done with conscious sedation. Patients' personal medical history may preclude conscious sedation, or their physiological makeup may rule out light sedation for even the most minimal procedure. Supporting clinical personnel should receive formal training in conscious sedation and should be familiar with all its requirements. Monitoring should include EKG, blood pressure, and pulse oximetry.

> SOME PATIENTS ARE NOT CANDIDATES FOR CONSCIOUS SEDATION, EVEN IF THE PROCEDURE THAT IS PRESCRIBED FOR THEM COULD BE DONE WITH CONSCIOUS SEDATION.

LOCAL ANESTHESIA

Local anesthesia involves simple infiltration of local anesthetic subcutaneously, submucosally, or near neurovascular bundles. Paracervical anesthesia for hysteroscopy and endometrial biopsy has been compared to placebo and found to reduce vasovagal responses and pain

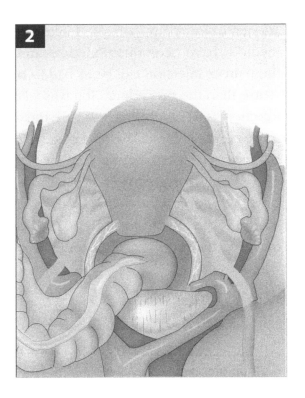

associated with the procedures. The innervation of the uterus is derived from the hypogastric and ovarian plexuses and from the third and fourth sacral nerves (Figure 2). The efferent fibers of the hypogastric plexus travel through the uterosacral ligaments.

The accurate placement of the anesthetic into the uterosacral ligaments will block most of the nerve fibers supplying the region of the internal cervical os. The paracervical or uterosacral block therefore can obliterate most of the pain sensations from cervical dilatation. A 1% Xylocaine solution is injected barely beneath the cervicovaginal mucosa at 5 o'clock and 7 o'clock position (Figure 3). Three to 4 cc of the anesthetic solution injected in each ligament is adequate for pain control. Infiltration methods have been questioned because the pain of injection can be as bad as or worse than the procedure. Intravascular injection and total dose of anesthetic must be considered. Topical anesthesia consisting of 2 mL of 2% mepivacaine injected transcervically into the uterine cavity was found to reduce vasovagal reactions but was not as effective in reducing the pain of the procedure.

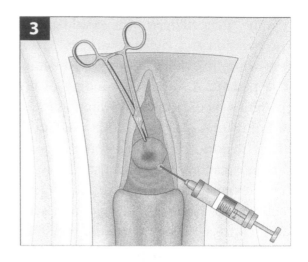

COMPLICATIONS OF DIAGNOSTIC HYSTEROSCOPY

The most commonly reported complication of diagnostic hysteroscopy is a vagovagal response from stimulation or stretching of the viscera. This response can be preemptively blocked with local anesthesia or treated by briefly stopping the procedure and/or treating with glycopyrrolate, or if unresponsive, with atropine. If CO_2 is used as a distension medium, pain under the shoulder from diaphragmatic irritation by the CO_2 can be more bothersome than the procedure itself. This can be alleviated with a Cox-2 inhibitor or other pain medication, but often just an explanation to the patient will suffice to allay anxiety about an unexpected area of pain. When using CO_2 as the distension medium, the most severe complication is a gas embolism, which, as explained earlier, can often be adequately treated if recognized early.

COMPLICATIONS OF OPERATIVE HYSTEROSCOPY

The best known complication from operative hysteroscopy is commonly described in the literature as the female TURP syndrome. Fluid overload and dilutional hyponatremia from absorption of fluid from open vessels, combined with a mechanical pressure augmentation, results in a potentially severe and possibly fatal condition. A triad of volume overload, dilutional hyponatremia, and hypo-osmolality, if unrecognized and untreated, can result in seizures, cerebral edema, and cardiorespiratory arrest.

Rapidly recognized as a potentially major problem with hysteroscopy, this triad has remarkable similarity to complications formerly described for transurethral resection of the prostate. This similarity was discovered the hard way, through unfortunate experiences.

Advances in distention media, technique, and equipment have led to a marked reduction in the incidence and severity of this complication. Keeping in mind the ever-present possibility of this complication leads to early detection and limited morbidity.

EVOLUTION OF HYPO-OSMOLAR HYPONATREMIA – THE FEMALE TURP SYNDROME

Hypo-osmolar hyponatremia with fluid overload is not unique to hysteroscopic procedures. Absorption of large amounts of fluid was first described in association with transurethral resection of the prostate. Unfortunately some deaths were reported during hysteroscopic surgery before it was realized that there was a striking similarity to the syndrome reported with TURP. The osmotic fluid gradient now favors movement of fluid into the interstitial compartment.

INCIDENCE

Fluid overload occurs in 0.2–6% of procedures. It has been defined as a fluid deficit reaching 2000 mL. This number is highly variable depending on the pre-existing condition of the patient. Hysteroscopic adhesiolysis, myomectomies, and resection of uterine septa have been reported in association with an increased incidence of fluid overload. Absorption of distension fluid

appears to depend on the duration of the resection and amount of tissue disruption, but also, and perhaps more importantly, on the pressure of the fluid. Fluid is absorbed from blood vessels that are disrupted in the uterus during the operation. There are reports indicating that the incidence of fluid absorption can be decreased by timing the surgery to the beginning of the menstrual cycle when decreased vascularity exists or to decrease vascularity chemically. A significant portion of fluid can also be absorbed through the peritoneal cavity from patent fallopian tubes. A 20% decrease in fluid absorption was found to occur in patients with prior tubal ligations. Pre-menopausal women are more susceptible to hyponatremia resulting in encephalopathy. One study reported that women have a 25 times greater incidence of permanent brain damage from hyponatremia as compared to men.

PATHOPHYSIOLOGY

As the fluid is absorbed, all elements of the blood are diluted and the intravascular volume is expanded. Hemodilution as well as dilution of electrolytes will occur to varying degrees. The patient's compensatory mechanisms and place on the Frank–Starling curve will determine when symptoms begin to appear. Initially as the load on the normal heart is increased, the heart will compensate by enlarging and increasing the force of contraction. Fluid in the vascular space enters the interstitium after 30–35 minutes as the dilution of plasma proteins favors the diffusion of fluid to the interstitium. As this fluid traverses into the interstitium, sodium will move with it, further complicating the developing hyponatremia (Figure 4). The particular symptoms that are manifested by the patient are a result of the final predominant imbalance of fluids and electrolytes, the surgical blood loss, the patient's medical status, and the anesthesia.

Regional anesthesia affords the advantage of an increased venous capacity from the sympathetic blockade and the advantage of cerebral monitoring from a semi-conscious patient. But regional anesthesia may not be feasible in some patients. There are no comparative studies to establish that regional anesthesia decreases the incidence of this syndrome. Symptoms may exist primarily due to predominant effects in the cardiovascular and central nervous systems or a combination of both systems. Each of these systems may be affected with or without hyponatremia.

THE EFFECTS OF FLUID OVERLOAD

Fluid overload in the cardiovascular system will result in peripheral edema, pulmonary edema, hypotension and congestive heart failure. The movement of fluid from the intravascular compartment to the interstitial compartment in the brain is responsible for the most life-threatening complications of the syn-

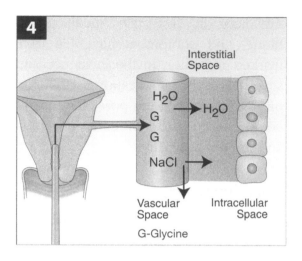

drome. As autoregulation is overcome, increasing cerebral edema decreases cerebral perfusion pressure. Both perfusion and adequate cell function, determined by electrolyte concentration can become problematic in this scenario. Complications of this syndrome include cerebral edema, seizures, possible herniation and death.

THE EFFECTS OF HYPONATREMIA

Hyponatremia is well tolerated if it occurs gradually. However this is not the case in this scenario. Symptoms may appear when the serum sodium is decreased below 130 mEq/L, although this range is considerable. Central nervous system effects occur below 120 mEq/L in most individuals. The earliest symptoms are restlessness and confusion followed by deterioration to seizures and loss of consciousness. The advantage of regional anesthesia is that these symptoms will be detected sooner in an awake patient.

CARDIOVASCULAR

The decrease in available sodium prevents adequate propagation of the action potential that exerts a negative inotropic effect on the myocardium, resulting in decreased response to the fluid increase that is being projected into the cardiovascular system. Electrocardiographic changes usually occur below 120 mEq/L. The action potential is reflected in the electrocardiogram as a widening of the QRS and ST segment elevation. If severe and untreated, ventricular tachycardia and fibrillation can occur.

SYMPTOMS IN THE CONSCIOUS PATIENT

- DYSPNEA
- SEDATION
- RESTLESSNESS
- CONFUSION
- CHEST PAIN
- NAUSEA AND VOMITING
- HEADACHE
- BLURRED VISION

OTHER EFFECTS

Hyperglycinemia may cause visual disturbances. Hyperammonemia can contribute to cerebral dysfunction. A high glucose can occur in both diabetics and non-diabetics.

THE VIGILANT OPERATING ROOM TEAM

Vigilance is actually the responsibility of everyone on the operating room team, not just the anesthesiologist. Judgments will be made on fluid estimates and serum sodium determinations. Many automated systems have been tried but none have been shown to have a greater accuracy. Communication between the surgeon, anesthesiologist and nursing staff is key to the most accurate estimate. Irrigation fluid should be assessed frequently. The prompt evaluation of electrolytes and volume status of the patient will help prevent the development of this syndrome. Surgical time should not be allowed to go beyond 60–90 minutes.

Ananthanarayan's suggested regime for fluid management is to measure serum electrolytes after a 500cc deficit. Administer Lasix after a 1000cc deficit. Terminate the procedure if serum sodium is significantly lowered or the deficit reaches 2000cc.

The anesthesiologist's index of suspicion must be high and diagnostic skills keen. A diligent record of the fluid balance must be recorded. This responsibility is a cooperative effort of the entire surgical team and not only the anesthesiologist. Fluid estimates are prone to human error and for this reason automated systems have been developed (See Chapter 2 on Instruments). These systems are not error free and are costly so estimates are by far the most com-

Chapter 4

46 | CHOICE OF ANESTHESIA ....

mon system in use today. While a diligent record of fluid balance should be attempted, one study demonstrated the operating room staff's gross errors in the estimation of fluid on the floor by a factor of 56%–67%. Suction canisters were sometimes found to be inaccurate. Even the amount of fluid in the irrigation bag can be 62–125 mL more than indicated on the bag. However an estimate is made, it is only an estimate, and the ultimate decision rests on the clinical and laboratory assessment of the patient.

The TURP syndrome, the laboratory measured relative serum sodium, does not always reflect the amount of fluid absorbed. Other factors including the stress of surgery are well known to release ADH, which will reduce the elimination of water and contribute to fluid overload. Since internal disruption of vessels from surgery, blood loss, and amount of fluid absorbed can only be estimated, clinical judgment along with laboratory values must suffice. Most often the patient will be asleep, and initial signs of confusion, agitation, irritability, and headache are symptoms that will manifest only in the recovery room. Likewise, nausea and vomiting that may occur after the absorption of 1000 mL of distension medium will not be seen during general anesthesia. Furthermore, the patient's medical condition can be a large factor in the timing of the development of symptoms. Decompensation may occur in the operating room or may not be manifested

until the patient is in the recovery room. Prompt recognition of signs and symptoms and rapid initiation of treatment will decrease morbidity significantly.

TREATMENT

Early signs of hypo-osmolar hyponatremia will initially manifest as fluid overload alone. Initially the blood pressure and heart rate will increase as the body attempts to accommodate the extra fluid. The patient's medical condition will determine to what extent symptoms develop. Oxygenation may decrease and in a great majority of cases only a diuretic and oxygen will be all that is necessary.

Serum electrolytes should be drawn to determine the trend of decline or stability in serum levels. Mild hyponatremia should rectify with diuretics and fluid restriction.

Treatment is supportive and corrective. At the first suspicion of the diagnosis, the operation should be terminated. If the patient is still intubated, optimizing oxygenation and ventilation by increasing the percentage of inspired oxygen and beginning ascending levels of positive end expiratory pressure, tempered by what the patient's cardiovascular system can tolerate, will improve oxygenation and help to oppose further fluid movement into the aveoli. Invasive monitoring including a Swan–Ganz catheter and arterial line may be necessary in severe cases to monitor the patient's condition.

If the syndrome first manifests in the recovery room, intubation may be necessary to adequately oxygenate the patient. A chest x-ray should be ordered and serial electrolytes as well as hourly urine output should be monitored at frequent intervals. Ventilation should continue until the patient is responsive, maintains adequate oxygenation and blood pressure, and meets the customary criteria to be extubated.

The initial response to quickly correct electrolytes must be avoided. The administration of hypertonic saline is not always indicated and is based on the severity of symptoms. Some patients are not symptomatic even with very low sodium. One study reports that 66% of TURP patients improved on diuretics and fluid restriction alone. These patients had a low sodium but a near normal osmolar gap. The serum sodium must be interpreted in light of the total serum osmolality. If both are low, hypertonic saline may be indicated for slow infusion.

The rate and amount of correction of serum sodium are controversial. If correction is too slow, the patient could worsen, and too fast correction has been implicated in causing central pontine demyelination. Sodium should not be corrected more than 1–2 mol/L/hr over the first few hours and slowed in subsequent hours. One or two ampules of sodium bicarbonate (50 mmol) may be all that is necessary and could be instituted prior to hypertonic saline. If hypertonic saline is begun, a 3%–5% solution of 200–500 mL over 4 hrs should be run slowly.

The goal of administration should be for only a partial correction guided by improvement in symptoms. It should be remembered that if saline is administered the intravascular load will initially be increased. The patient's status may worsen if already in fluid overload status or borderline on the Starling curve. A diuretic will need to be administered concurrently in that instance. Awareness of this syndrome and early recognition and prompt initiation of treatment measures have lead to a great reduction in morbidity and increased safety of this procedure.

SUMMARY

Hysteroscopy has an ever-widening scope of applications. Diagnostic hysteroscopy has much less risk associated with it, although precautions must be taken to avoid undue sedation and morbidity. Surgical therapeutic hysteroscopy has the potential for significant morbidity and even mortality. Although perforation is the most common complication, the triad of fluid overload, hyponatremia, and hypo-osmolality can result in the female TURP syndrome. A high index of suspicion with diligent monitoring and attention to fluid deficit will give the earliest indication of impending morbidity. Prompt diagnosis and pertinent treatment are necessary for optimal patient outcome.

Chapter 4

48 | CHOICE OF ANESTHESIA ···

SUGGESTED READING:

Ananthanarayan C, Paek W, Rolbin SH, et al. Hysteroscopy and anesthesia.
Can J Anaesth 1996;43:56-64

Arieff AI, Ayus JC. Treatment of symptomatic hyponatremia: Neither haste nor waste.
Crit Care Med 1991;19:748-51

Boyd HR, Stanley C. Sources of error when tracking irrigation fluids during hysteroscopic
procedures. J Am Assoc Gynecol Laparosc 2000;7(4):472-6

Cicinelli E, Didonna T, Fiore G, Parisi C, Matteo MG, Castrovilli G. Topical anesthesia for
hysteroscopy in postmenopausal women. J Am Assoc Gynecol Laparosc 1996;4(1):9-12

Cicinelli E, Dodonna T, Schonauer LM, Stragapede S, Falco N, Pansini N. Paracervical anesthesia for hysteroscopy and endometrial biopsy in postmenopausal women. A randomized,
double-blind, placebo-controlled study. J Reprod Med 1998;43(12):1014-8

Clark L. Anesthesia in Laparoscopy. In: A Practical Manual of Laparoscopy: A Clinical
Cookbook. Pasic R, Levine RL (eds). New York: Parthenon Publishers Group,
2002, pp 37-54

Cooper JM, Brady RM. Intraoperative and early postoperative complications of operative
hysteroscopy. Obstet Gynecol Clin North Am 2000;27(2):347-66

Gonzales R, Brensilver JM, Rovinsky JJ. Posthysteroscopic hyponatremia.
Am J Kidney Dis 1994;23:735-8

Hong JY, Oh JI, Kim SM. Comparison of sevoflurane-nitrous oxide and target-controlled
propofol with fentanyl anesthesia for hysteroscopy. Yonsei Med J 2002;43(4):420-6

Jansen FW, Vredevoogd CB, van Ulzen K, et al. Complications of hysteroscopy:
A prospective multicentre study. Obstet Gynecol 2000;96:266-70

Murdoch JA, Gan TJ. Anesthesia for hysteroscopy. Anesthesiol Clin North America
2001;19(1):125-40 (Review)

Mushambi MC, Williamson K. Anaesthetic considerations for hysteroscopic surgery.
Best Pract Res Clin Anaesthesiol 2002;16(1):35-52

Probst AM, Liberman RF, Harlow BL, Ginsburg ES. Complications of hysteroscopic surgery: Predicting patients at risk. Obstet Gynecol 2000;96:517-20

Sherlock S, Shearer WA, Buist M, et al. Carbon dioxide embolism following diagnostic hysteroscopy. Anaesth Intens Care 1998;26:674-6

ELECTROSURGERY IN THE UTERUS

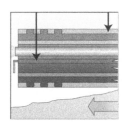 *Malcolm G. Munro, M.D.*

INTRODUCTION

Operative hysteroscopy is used to dissect, resect, or ablate tissue within or adjacent to the endometrial cavity. Cup forceps are effective for targeted biopsy and mechanical scissors can be used for adhesions and removal of a septum occasionally. However, most therapeutic procedures require the use of an energy source transmitted to the endometrial cavity. Although lasers were the first energy sources used, electrosurgery provided the best combination of effectiveness, efficiency, and acceptable cost. Electrosurgery refers to the application of radiofrequency (RF) alternating current to elevate intracellular temperature resulting in tissue vaporization or coagulation. The uterine environment and the incumbent requirement to operate in a fluid environment present a number of challenges both to surgeons and to the manufacturers of hysteroscopic surgical equipment. The surgeon should be familiar with electrical principles as they apply to the equipment, thus ensuring that the desired tissue effect is achieved and risks of complications are minimized.

Chapter 5

50 | ELECTROSURGERY IN THE UTERUS . . . .

FUNDAMENTALS

In electrosurgery, electrical energy is converted in the tissue to thermal energy. If the cell heats rapidly, beyond the boiling point of water, the cellular contents turn to steam and rapidly expand, rupturing the cell wall in a process called vaporization. If the intracellular temperature is sharply elevated, but remains below the boiling point of water, the intracellular water is lost by dehydration. Ultimately, this results in desiccation and the molecular bonds of the cell are broken then haphazardly reformed when the tissue cools. A homogeneous coagulum results in a process called coagulation. The type of tissue effect is determined by a number of electrical properties as well as factors such as tissue exposure time, the size and shape of the electrode, and the relationship of the electrode to the target tissue.

ELECTROSURGICAL CIRCUITS

RF electrosurgery requires the formation of a circuit for the passage of electrons that includes the electrodes, the patient, the electrosurgical generator or unit (ESU) and the connecting wires. In the "monopolar" system, the active electrode is within the endometrial cavity near the target tissue, while the second, dispersive electrode is positioned elsewhere on the patient, typically the thigh. As a result, much of the patient is interposed between the two electrodes. The "bipolar" system is designed so that

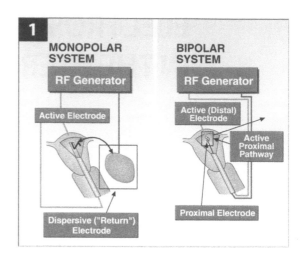

both the distal or active and the proximal electrode are within the endometrial cavity, reducing patient exposure to electrical current to the tissue immediately in the target area. This configuration allows for enough reduction in impedance to make function in physiologic solutions possible (Figure 1). While all RF electrosurgery requires two electrodes, bipolar instruments are designed to contain both electrodes. This circumstance limits the portion of the patient involved in the circuit to the tissue that is near to or interposed between the two electrodes. Monopolar instruments are designed with only one electrode for concentrating the current and generating the tissue effect, while the other electrode is placed remotely on the patient. While many call this electrode a "return" electrode, the appropriate name is the dispersive electrode since it acts as a conduit for the same number of moving electrons. However, by diluting them over a much wider area it prevents the occurrence of a local thermal effect. Because of this configuration, the circuit includes the whole patient, a circumstance that provides a greater opportunity for current to be diverted to undesirable locations.

FUNDAMENTALS OF ELECTRICITY

The three interacting properties of electricity that are fundamental to understanding RF electrosurgery are current (I), voltage (V), and impedance or resistance (R). Current, propagated by ionic effects, is a measure of the electron movement past a point in the circuit in a given period of time. It is measured in amperes. Voltage describes the electromotive pressure with which the electrons are pushed through the tissue. It is measured in volts. Resistance is measured in ohms, and is a reflection of the difficulty a given substance (e.g., tissue) presents to the passage of electrons. The term resistance is generally reserved for direct current while, for alternating current, the term impedance is used.

In a given circuit, these properties are related by Ohm's Law: $I = V/R$. An effective hydraulic analogy explaining these properties has been designed by Roger Odell. Voltage is in essence electrical pressure, similar to the pressure developed on the contents of a water tower, which can be increased by raising the level of the tower. When voltage increases, the current increases just as

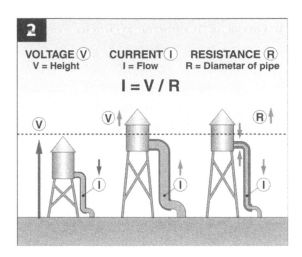

the flow of water increases through the spigot of the water tower. Tissue impedance, if increased, impedes the flow of electrons (current) just as narrowing the diameter of the spigot reduces the flow of water from the water tower (Figure 2). The height of the water tower creates the pressure (voltage) exerted upon the water in the outflow pipe. The water passes through the pipe (flow of current) which, if widened, would increase flow (decreased resistance), and if narrowed would restrict flow (higher resistance). Power (W), the capacity to do work per unit time, is a product of current and voltage and is measured in watts ($W = V \times I$). If Ohm's Law is used to create a substitution for current [$W = V \times (V/R)$], then wattage can be expressed in another way ($W = V2/R$).

These relationships are helpful in explaining a number of features of electrosurgery. For example, the ratio of voltage to current (V/I) is largely responsible for the differing effects on tissue, given similar electrode size and shape as well as tissue exposure time. In general, the "pressure" of increased voltage enhances the ability of the current to arc from the electrode to tissue. In addition, this pressure forces more energy into the tissue, a circumstance that fosters a greater degree of thermal injury. The power equation ($W = V^2/R$) shows how a standard electrosurgical generator, at a given output in watts, will diminish the output voltage if the tissue resistance increases. This helps to explain how the cutting or coagulating characteristics of an electrode may change as tissues with different resistance are encountered.

RF ELECTROSURGICAL GENERATORS AND WAVEFORMS

The ESU converts a 60 cycle per second (60 Hertz or Hz) low voltage alternating current into higher voltage radiofrequency (300 kHz to 3.0 MHz) current. This current is then produced either continuously or intermittently with cyclically variable voltage. If such an output is connected to an oscilloscope, it is displayed as a waveform. RF output cyclically varies voltage about 500,000 times per second by changing (alternating) the polarity of the electrodes. The oscillating output therefore results in oscillating intracellular anions and cations. This is preferable to directional current flow that is seen only in direct current (DC) circuits (Figure 3). The wave is generally symmetrical

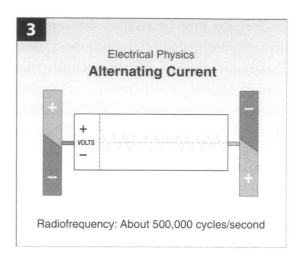

above and below "0" volts reflecting the nature of an alternating current, oscillating back and forth at the output frequency of the generator instead of flowing in one direction. The peak voltage generated is depicted by the distance from the baseline to the apex of the wave.

The output labelled 'cut' provides a continuous low voltage waveform. As it is seen on the oscilloscope, the waveform is typically that of a sinewave, reflecting the continuously alternating polarity of RF current. The so-called 'coagulation' mode is an interrupted, dampened, and relatively high voltage waveform. The generator can produce differing waveforms and modulate the current to allow the creation of different tissue effects. A term used to describe output modulation is "duty cycle" which describes the percentage of time that the circuit is on. For example, for the high voltage output usually called "coagulation", the duty cycle is typically about

6%, as current is off 94% of the time. At the opposite side of the spectrum is the "pure cut" output which, by virtue of being continuous, has a duty cycle of 100%. The so-called "blend" outputs are actually low voltage cut outputs that are modulated with a duty cycle of less than 100% but generally greater than 50%. By reducing the duty cycle, the voltage increases, a circumstance that is designed to result in greater collateral thermal damage along the line of vaporization or transection (Figure 4). Blended currents were formerly created by combining the two types of waveforms described above. However, all modern ESUs create their 'blended' currents by producing interrupted or modulated versions of the 'cut' waveforms. When the current is interrupted, and wattage is held constant, the generator increases the voltage of the output (W = V x I). In the water tower analogy, this is equivalent to elevating the level of the tower while intermittently turning the water flow on and off at the tap. The increased pressure afforded by the height of the tower allows a greater amount of water to flow along the pipe per unit time. Typically it is possible for the operator to vary the effect by selecting from a number of blend modes that vary the duty cycle from, for example, 80% (Blend 1) to 50% (Blend 3). As the duty cycle diminishes, the peak voltage increases, a factor that allows more collateral thermal damage and a consequently greater hemostatic effect.

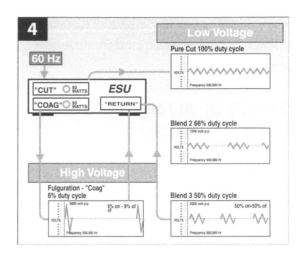

It is important to realize that all generators are not created equally. The duty cycles of the various "blend" modes vary from machine to machine. The peak voltages generated in any of the modes may vary significantly depending, in part, on the purpose for which the machine was designed. For example, machines designed for operating room use generally provide peak voltages for the continuous and blended waveforms significantly higher than machines designed for outpatient loop electrosurgical excision of the cervix. This is largely because the operating room machines are designed to deal with tissue that has high impedance. The tradeoff is that thermal injury will be greater with the increased voltage.

Most ESUs designed for operating room use have the capability of providing bipolar current. Modern generators only provide a continuous waveform, identical to the 'cut' waveform, even though bipolar devices are not really capable of a cutting effect. The reasons for this will be explained in subsequent sections.

EFFECT OF ALTERNATING CURRENT ON CELLS

We alluded to the fact that RF electricity may be used to either cut or vaporize cells and tissue, depending upon the intracellular temperature achieved. In this section the mechanism by which these effects occur will be explained.

Cells contain both cations and anions. The former are small, positively charged particles like sodium and potassium while the latter include large, negatively charged protein molecules. When an RF alternating current is applied across the cell, the rapidly changing polarity of the current causes these cations and anions to equally oscillate rapidly within the cytoplasm. This essentially represents a conversion of electromagnetic energy to mechanical energy. However, the friction caused by molecular oscillation immediately induces another energy conversion, that of mechanical energy to thermal energy, a conversion that elevates the intracellular temperature. If enough energy is transmitted to the cell to heat it to 70–90°C, the water changes to water vapor leaving the cell (desiccation) and protein bonds broken to then reform creating an amorphous proteinaceous tissue (coagulation) (Figure 5). As the

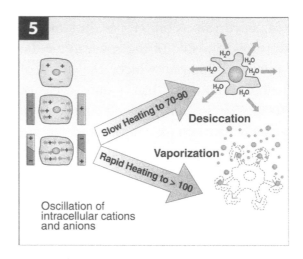

Oscillation of intracellular cations and anions

temperature rises, intracellular water is lost by dehydration. If the intracellular temperature reaches about 70°–90°, protein denaturation occurs as molecular bonds break down. The end point of dehydration is cellular desiccation while the molecular bonds reform in an interlaced but haphazard fashion that creates a homogeneous proteinaceous tissue in a process called coagulation. Cellular vaporization occurs if there is adequate energy to rapidly elevate the temperature beyond 100°. In such circumstances the intracellular water boils and the subsequent formation of steam and intracellular expansion results in explosive vaporization of the cell (Figure 5). It is suspected that the explosive force results in acoustical vibrations that contribute to the cutting effect through the tissue. The gases produced as a result of this process of vaporization largely comprise hydrogen (about 50%) as well as carbon dioxide and carbon monoxide as well as smaller amounts of other organic substances.

The frequency of the current is key to establishing the effect and in eliminating some undesirable effects on nerve and muscle including myocardium. This is because low frequency alternating current has a different effect on the cell. If the frequency is below 30 kHz but above 20 Hz it will predictably cause a Faradic effect – the depolarization of muscles and nerves resulting in fasciculation and pain. With radiofrequency current the cell's positive and negative ions vacillate so rapidly that depolarization does not occur. Despite these theoretical considerations, radiofrequency alternating current up to 1 MHz can cause neuromuscular stimulation. The exact reasons for such stimulation are not known but could include the influence of stray, lower frequency arcs to tissue or rectification – the conversion of alternating current to direct current.

TISSUE EFFECTS OF ELECTROSURGERY

Electrosurgery may be used either to vaporize or coagulate tissue. If vaporization is extended in a linear fashion, cutting occurs. To a greater or lesser extent, a zone of coagulation will be created adjacent to any electrosurgical incision or other zone of vaporization. The tissue effects depend upon a number of factors including the power, tissue impedance, the waveform, the distending media, the shape and size of the electrode and its proximity to tissue, i.e., contact or non-contact.

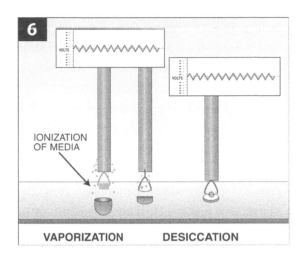

Critical to the understanding of tissue effects is the concept of current or power density (Figure 6). The power density is the total wattage striking the tissue per unit area of the electrode or current in contact with that tissue. Given equal power outputs, power density is largely determined by the shape and size of the electrode and by its relationship to the tissue, i.e., contact vs. non-contact. An electrode with a small surface area such as resection loop, and particularly if held near to but not in contact with the tissue, will concentrate current so that the point of impact on tissue is very narrow and the power density high. This allows for a very localized focusing of energy with consequent rapid elevation of cellular temperature and the creation of a narrow zone of vaporization. Given the same power, a wider, larger electrode such as a ball or barrel held in contact with tissue, will dilute the power density, thereby transmitting the same amount of energy to a larger volume of tissue. This is a circumstance that prevents rapid elevation of intracellular temperature. Instead the temperature rises more slowly, not reaching the boiling point of water, but is enough to cause protein coagulation and desiccation. The extreme of power density reduction is manifest in the dispersive electrode. Remember that the dispersive electrode transmits the same power, but its surface area is so large that it dissipates the current to the point that no significant temperature elevation occurs and, consequently, there is no significant tissue effect.

CUTTING

Linear vaporization (cutting) of tissue is best achieved with a continuous or near continuous, monopolar, low voltage output, using a pointed or a thin needle or loop shaped electrode held near but not in contact with the tissue. The generator is activated, allowing the thin electrode to concentrate the current at its tip, which, if sufficient, ionizes the medium around it forming a sort of plasma cloud. Provided the voltage is adequate, and the electrode is near to the tissue, the ionized medium becomes part of the circuit and the current then arcs to the nearby tissue, rapidly elevating the intracellular temperature resulting in vaporization. The steam from vaporization contains ions that contribute to the existing ionized medium, reducing the impedance between the electrode and tissue, thereby facilitating continued propagation of the current. As the electrode is advanced, an incision is fashioned as continued arcing and vaporization of the underlying tissue maintain the process. The continuous nature of the current ensures a continuous production of steam (the steam "envelope") that in turn facilitates the localized targeting of the impact site of the current on the tissue. Modulated currents are more likely to lose the steam envelope and function far less efficiently, and with greater current dispersion. Furthermore, because the voltage is low and the current dissipates rapidly towards the dispersive electrode, the thermal damage beside the cut is minimal provided appropriate equipment and surgical technique are used.

The actual depth of coagulation injury incurred during linear vaporization is dependent upon a number of factors including power output, electrode size and shape, waveform and peak voltage, and the speed and skill of the surgeon. Consequently, descriptions of the depth of coagulation injury should take the existence of such variables into consideration. While the minimum depth of thermal injury has been described as low as a few microns, more typical reported endomyometrial injury studies suggest about 0.5 to 1.5 mm.

BULK VAPORIZATION

As its name implies, bulk vaporization refers to the use of RF techniques to remove relatively large masses of tissue by electrosurgical vaporization. The technique requires a large electrode and the process is facilitated if the surface of the electrode is grooved or spiked creating localized areas where power or current can concentrate, often called edge density. With adequate power, the bulk-vaporizing electrode will function like an array of small loop electrodes simultaneously vaporizing adjacent areas of tissue resulting in the rapid vaporization of tissue mass. To achieve the required power, the ESU is set at three to four times the power than is the case for linear vaporization with loop or needle electrodes. There is a substantial amount of gas produced by the bulk vaporization of such large masses of tissue.

DESICCATION/COAGULATION

Coagulation is generally used to depict one or more of a number of related processes where the cell is dehydrated and the protein is denatured but not destroyed by the thermal energy. When an electrode is placed in contact with the tissue, all the energy is available for conversion to heat. Furthermore, the relatively large contact area of a ball or barrel reduces the power density, preventing elevation of the intracellular temperature to 100°, thereby allowing desiccation and coagulation to occur.

Although any waveform may be used to create tissue coagulation, the cutting and blended outputs are preferred to the labeled "coagulation" mode. The interrupted nature of the "coagulation" current may cause an uneven amount of protein bonding, theoretically reducing the homogeneity of the tissue effect. Early coagulation of the superficial layers of the tissue could result in increased impedance, reducing further transmission of current to the deeper layers. Despite these theoretical concerns, coagulation waveforms may be adequately effective within the endometrial cavity for the purposes of tissue coagulation. However, it is clear that high voltage outputs damage electrodes more quickly and that the risk of capacitative coupling, to be discussed later in this chapter, is higher with coagulation outputs. Such coupling may be associated with increased risks of unintended current diversion and vaginal, and vulvar burns from an activated external sheath. As a result, it would seem prudent to eliminate or minimize the use of this current during operative hysteroscopy.

As a result of these considerations, coagulation should be performed with an electrode having a relatively large surface area, using the 'cutting' or 'blended' waveforms. If a blood vessel is to be coagulated, it should be first coapted by compressing it with a large electrode then activating the generator using suitable low voltage current.

FULGURATION

Fulguration, also known as spray coagulation or black coagulation, is a process in which the tissue is superficially carbonized by repeated high voltage electrosurgical arcs that quickly elevate the temperature to 200° or more. This process is achieved by spraying energy onto tissue using an interrupted high voltage current with a dampened or modulated waveform – the "coagulation" output (Figure 6). The nature of hysteroscopic electrosurgery and the fluid media in which it is practiced renders the mechanisms involved in fulguration difficult if not impossible to achieve, leaving it as a technique that may be applied at either open or laparoscopic surgery.

INSTRUMENTATION

Electrosurgical generators and hysteroscopic instrumentation, including the design and basic function of the uterine resectoscope, have been described in detail in Chapter 2. In this chapter, the electrode selection and generator settings will be discussed in more detail.

COAGULATION/DESICCATION ELECTRODES

There exists a variety of rolling electrode shapes including ball, barrel, and ellipsoid, as well as large caliber loops, each of which allows the surgeon to achieve the desired effect while in contact with the tissue surface (Figure 7). The depth of coagulation achieved with a given electrode is dependent upon a

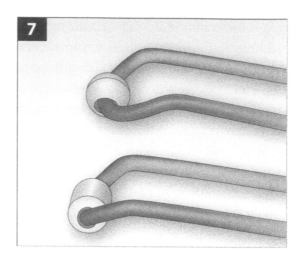

number of variables including ESU factors such as waveform and power setting; electrode-related issues such as size, shape, and cleanliness; technique-based factors such as tissue exposure time (speed of the electrode) and the amount of pressure applied while moving the device; and tissue-related features such as endometrial thickness and the variations in tissue impedance related to the presence or absence of desiccation created by previous passes of the device.

There is considerable controversy regarding the best waveform for the creation of deep coagulation within the endometrial cavity. Although there is clear evidence that low voltage continuous ("cut") current is preferable for coaptation of blood vessels or fallopian tubes at laparoscopy or laparotomy, there is little evidence upon which a case can be made for either for hysteroscopic electrosurgery. For example, there have been no studies comparing clinical outcomes associated with the two types of output, and there is even a paucity of in vitro information. However, theoretically at least, wave-forms and other settings and techniques that result in slower heating of tissue are more likely to result in deep and homogenous tissue penetration. Furthermore, as will be described in the section of this chapter on complications, there exists an evolving rationale to avoid the use of high voltage outputs ("coag") because of the increased risk of capacitative coupling. Regardless of the output selected, the surgeon should strive to move the electrode in a linear fashion at a constant and slow pace all the while visualizing the continuous stream of bubbles emanating from the desiccating tissue and the trailing symmetrical coagulated tissue.

CUTTING ELECTRODES

Loop electrodes are made with a curved wire and can resect tissue by virtue of the zone of high power density created along their narrow surface area (Figure 8). Unlike desiccation, linear vaporization, or cutting, is initiated by near-contact activation of the electrode, which, provided the generator settings are appropriate (low voltage current 60–80 W on most generators), results in arcing of current to tissue and resultant focused cellular vaporization. With the establishment of the steam envelope (often called plasma cloud) the electrode can be withdrawn toward the

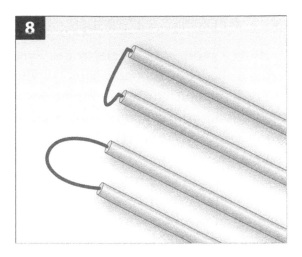

operator as the tissue is cut by vaporization, not by mechanical means. In effect, the surgeon should conceptualize the energy leading the electrode through the tissue, rather than the perception that a hot electrode cuts by contact. Indeed, with tissue contact, desiccation may predominate, the steam envelope diminishes or disappears, and the vaporization effect will diminish or cease.

If a greater degree of desiccation is desired along the edge of an electrosurgical incision, the low voltage waveform can be modulated, and voltage slightly increased using the so-called blended waveforms. These waveforms produce ample energy for linear vaporization yet create a slightly thicker zone of collateral tissue coagulation that may improve hemostasis, a feature useful for hysteroscopic myomectomy or endometrial resection.

BULK VAPORIZING ELECTRODES

Bulk vaporization electrodes are often called by the trade name of the original manufacturer – Vaportrodes. Concentration of current at the edge of an electrode is a natural electrical phenomenon. Grooved or spiked barrel-shaped electrodes possess a number of these edges, which essentially function like an array of narrow caliber electrodes, each with the ability to vaporize nearby tissue (Figure 9). The resulting aggregation of vapor tracks merge into one as the electrode is drawn through tissue ablating large volumes of tissue. Such a technique effectively vaporizes leiomyomas dramatically reducing the need to remove the resectoscope for removal of resected tissue. There is also evidence that bulk vaporization may be a superior technique for endometrial ablation when compared to endometrial resection, largely because of the increased amount of collateral desiccation in the remaining endometrium when compared to that associated with endometrial resection. This zone of desiccation is the suggested explanation for the observed reduction in systemic absorption of distension media. However the use of this technique should be avoided at the corneal areas and the isthmus to reduce the risk of electrosurgical perforation of the uterus. Because several zones of high current density must be created to achieve this effect, the power requirements are several times higher for this type of elec-

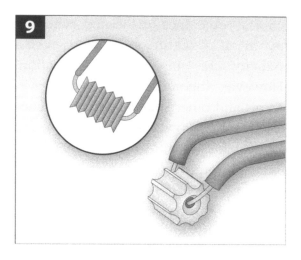

trode. For example, with a Valleylab Force F/X electrode settings of 200–220 watts are necessary; for some ESUs with lower peak voltage, higher settings may be necessary for an optimal effect.

BIPOLAR ELECTRODES

The potential perils of hyponatremic and hypo-osmolar distension media are discussed in Chapters 4 and 20. Excessive intravasation of such media results in complications that include hyponatremia, hypo-osmolality, cerebral edema, and death. Such complications were the major incentive behind the development and introduction of bipolar hysteroscopic electrodes that can function effectively in physiological solutions.

Available bipolar systems (Versapoint™ System, Gynecare Division of Ethicon Inc, Somerville, NJ; PK Saline TUR Gyrus Medical, Maple Grove MN) comprise a dedicated bipolar ESU that can be connected to one of three 36 cm long flexible coaxial catheters narrow enough to be passed through the 5-Fr working channel of an operating hysteroscope. The distal or tissue interface end of the catheter contains two electrodes separated by a ceramic insulator (Figure 10). The most distal of these electrodes is the active electrode while the proximally located electrode functions only to complete the circuit. Note that this component of the instrument does not necessarily function as a dispersive electrode, nor is it an electrode that is designed to create a tissue effect. The active electrode is available in a variety of compositions and shapes that result in a spectrum of tissue effects. The ball tip is for precise vaporization with limited desiccation, and the spring tip is designed as a type of bulk vaporizing electrode. The braided tip is a cutting device for resection and morcellation. Given the small caliber of these electrode tipped catheters, their use is limited to polypectomy, adhesiolysis, and vaporization or morcellation of smaller submucous myomata. Note that these electrodes are not designed to be used with a utcrinc resectoscope nor can they be used with any other ESUs. The same company has developed a resectoscope that appears and functions like a monopolar-based system (Versapoint™ Resectoscope) and can be used with specially configured loop and bulk vaporizing electrodes that function based on principles similar to those elucidated above (Figure 11). As

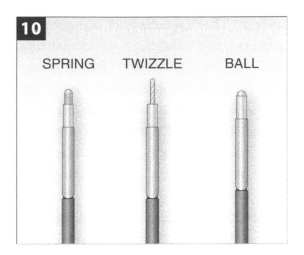

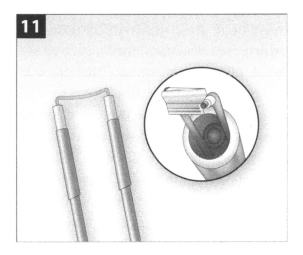

with the narrow caliber Versapoint™ System, resectoscope and electrodes can be used only with the dedicated ESU made by the manufacturer.

CREATING TISSUE EFFECTS IN FLUID MEDIA

Establishment and maintenance of an electrosurgical tissue effect requires that the desired power density be maintained. The intrauterine environment presents the challenge of establishing and maintaining the effect in the context of a fluid medium. Because electrolyte-containing distention media such as saline are effective conductors, monopolar instrumentation does not function in these fluids. If attempted, the electrolyte rich medium acts as a conductor that functionally enlarges the electrode's surface area, thereby dramatically reducing power density. Consequently, for monopolar instrumentation, it is necessary to use electrolyte free distention media such as sorbitol, glycine, or mannitol that are non-conductive and are insulators. In such circumstances, an activated electrode can maintain its power density as well as the electrosurgical effect following ionization of the media between electrode and tissue and the establishment of a vaporpocket largely comprising the steam and organic products of cellular vaporization (Figure 12). These products, almost invisible in the laparoscopic and open surgery environments, create bubbles in the endometrial cavity during operative hysteroscopy. It is known that these bubbles largely comprise hydrogen, carbon monoxide, and carbon dioxide, each of which is highly soluble in blood. Consequently, should these products enter the systemic circulation (as they often do) they dissolve in blood and do not present a cause for concern for the patient.

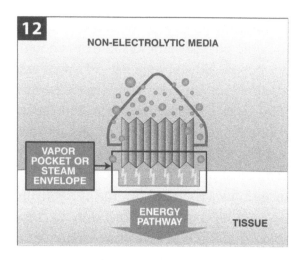

The relatively non-conductive nature of these distension media increase impedance, requiring, at least initially, that voltage in the circuit be higher. Consequently, the most effective ESUs are those that produce outputs with higher peak voltage. This is especially true for bulk vaporization where the generator is challenged with developing an extremely high current density over a relatively large electrode surface area. Such voltage requirements are less important for the initiation and maintenance of tissue coagulation.

The recently developed bipolar systems that can function in electrolyte rich environments were discussed previously. To function properly, both electrodes must be immersed in the isotonic saline media which itself becomes a part of the electrical circuit (Figure 13). Although high current density is developed on the proximal electrode, only the distal electrode is intended for tissue interaction. When the ESU is activated, and RF current with its alternating voltage is applied between the distal (active) and proximal electrodes, the intervening resistance of the saline is overcome as the intervening fluid media is ionized and the circuit is completed. The exact mechanisms by which tissue effects are generated remain unclear, but some hypotheses can be made. The local oscillation of the fluid media creates local heat, and, taken to an extreme, steam that forms a vaporpocket with internally low impedance focused around the distal or active electrode. When the active electrode is brought in proximity to the target tissue, the products of tissue vaporization are added to this vaporpocket. This pocket and adjacent ionized media then function as a low impedance pathway from the tissue to the active electrode to the proximal electrode and serves to effectively channel the current into the tissue by preventing dispersion into the surrounding electrolyte-rich distention medium. The Versapoint system has a dessicate (DES) mode in which the generator increases the temperature of the saline just short of the boiling point, but the impedance in the circuit is low, both at the active electrode tissue interface (where there is contact) and between the proximal and active electrodes where the local impedance of the heated saline is low enough to allow completion of the circuit.

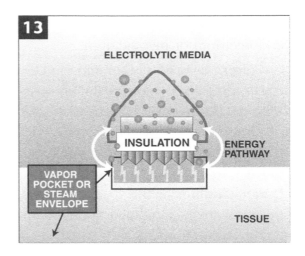

COMPLICATIONS

The major complications of intrauterine RF electrosurgery relate to uterine perforation and current diversion, the latter only related to the use of monopolar instrumentation.

Uterine perforation with an active electrode cannot occur unless the operator moves the electrode away from the tip of the hysteroscope or resectoscope while it is activated. In this way, it is possible both to perforate the uterus and to damage structures and viscera that surround the uterus in the pelvis, including bowel, ureter, bladder, and blood vessels. Due to the possibility of this type of perforation, the activated electrodes should not be moved forward. The exceptions to this rule are the division of a uterine septum and bulk vaporization of myomas particularly in fundal locations. Consequently, perhaps a more tenable rule would be to avoid any forward movement of an activated electrode while in the endometrium or myometrium.

Current diversion is common in electrosurgery with monopolar systems. When such diverted current is focused on tissue outside the target area, complications may occur, most commonly burns to the vagina or vulva. Understanding the mechanisms involved in such complications is the key to avoiding them.

Radiofrequency energy can be transferred from one circuit to another by direct contact (direct coupling) or without such contact (capacitive coupling), the latter is related to the existence of an energy field around any circuit. Even in the normal monopolar resectoscope, with an electrode with intact insulation, capacitive coupling occurs from the active electrode to the internal sheath and telescope, and then to the external sheath in all instances of electrode activation (Figure 14). Even more transmission might occur if direct coupling occurs from the electrode to the internal sheath or telescope to start the chain. However the amount of energy so transmitted, provided there is an intimate contact of the external sheath with the surrounding cervix, the circuit will be completed with the dispersive electrode without the creation of an area of high current density where an undesirable burn could occur. If the intimate relationship of the external sheath is lost, and replaced by a less extensive contact with the vagina or vulva, the scenario

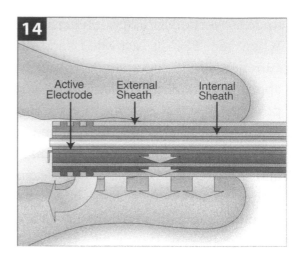

for a high power (current) density zone and resultant burn can be created (Figure 15).

The above description summarizes the presumed mechanism for a growing series of vulvar and vaginal thermal injuries reported in conjunction with the use of uterine resectoscopes and monopolar electrodes. The explanation behind direct coupling is somewhat simple as it requires a breech in the insulation around the electrode and the flexing of the electrode to result in contact with the internal sheath or telescope – with capacitative coupling completing the circuit with the external sheath. However, many factors that increase the risk of capacitative coupling and decrease contact with the cervix are less well understood. Investigation in our laboratory has shown that, in simulated conditions, high voltage currents such as those that come from the "coagulation" side of ESUs more likely result in significant capacitative coupling to the external sheath than is the case for low voltage current, even at relatively high outputs. Capacitative coupling will more likely occur if the surgeon keeps the electrode continuously active while not in direct or near contact with tissue. It is thought that the reasons for diminishing the interface between external sheath and cervix might occur as a result of overdilation, or, especially keeping the electrode fully extended while the entire unit is withdrawn to treat areas in the lower uterine segment.

The following principles serve to reduce the risk of such injuries. First and foremost, the use of electrodes with damaged insulation should be avoided – consequently, a new electrode should be used for each case. It is probably safer to use voltage cutting current, minimizing or avoiding the use of high voltage "coagulation" outputs since such waveforms probably facilitate these complications. More importantly, the surgeon should strive to maintain intimate contact between the external sheath and the cervix by not

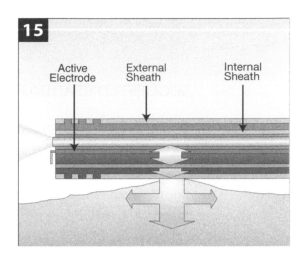

overdilating prior to starting the procedure and by keeping the external sheath fully in the cervix when operating. Finally, the electrode should be activated only when near or in contact with the target tissue.

Any metallic object including specula and cervical tenacula also can, following contact with the external sheath, serve to conduct current to locations in the vagina and vulva. Care should be taken to avoid contact of these instruments with the resectoscope.

Chapter 5

66 | **ELECTROSURGERY IN THE UTERUS** ....

SUGGESTED READING:

Bloomstone J, Chow CM, Isselbacher E, VanCott E, Isaacson KB. A pilot study examining the frequency and quantity of gas embolization during operative hysteroscopy using a monopolar resectoscope. J Am Assoc Gynecol Laparosc 2002;9(1):9-14

Brill AI. Energy systems for operative hysteroscopy. Obstet Gynecol Clin North Am 2000;27(2):317-26

Indman PD, Soderstrom RM. Depth of endometrial coagulation with the urologic resectoscope. J Reprod Med 1990;35(6):633-5

Isaacson KB, Olive DL. Operative hysteroscopy in physiologic distention media. J Am Assoc Gynecol Laparosc 1999;6(1):113-8

Munro MG, Brill AI, Ryan T, Ciarrocca S. Electrosurgery-induced generation of gases: comparison of in vitro rates of production using bipolar and monopolar electrodes. J Am Assoc Gynecol Laparosc 2003;10(2):252-9

Munro MG, Weisberg M, Rubinstein E. Gas and air embolization during hysteroscopic electrosurgical vaporization: comparison of gas generation using bipolar and monopolar electrodes in an experimental model. J Am Assoc Gynecol Laparosc 2001;8(4):488-94

Munro MG. Factors affecting capacitive current diversion with a uterine resectoscope: An in vitro study. J Am Assoc Gynecol Laparosc 2003;10(4):450-460

Vercellini P, Oldani S, Milesi M, Rossi M, Carinelli S, Crosignani PG. Endometrial ablation with a vaporizing electrode. I. Evaluation of in vivo effects. Acta Obstet Gynecol Scand 1998;77(6):683-7

Vercellini P, Oldani S, Yaylayan L, Zaina B, De Giorgi O, Crosignani PG. Randomized comparison of vaporizing electrode and cutting loop for endometrial ablation. Obstet Gynecol 1999;94(4):521-7

Vilos GA. Intrauterine surgery using a new coaxial bipolar electrode in normal saline solution (Versapoint): a pilot study. Fertil Steril 1999;72(4):740-3

Vilos GA, McCulloch S, Borg P, Zheng W, Denstedt J. Intended and stray radiofrequency electrical currents during resectoscopic surgery. J Am Assoc Gynecol Laparosc 2000;7(1):55-63

Vilos GA, Brown S, Graham G, McCulloch S, Borg P. Genital tract electrical burns during hysteroscopic endometrial ablation: report of 13 cases in the United States and Canada. J Am Assoc Gynecol Laparosc 2000;7(1):141-7

TECHNIQUES FOR DIAGNOSTIC HYSTEROSCOPY, HYSTEROSCOPIC RESECTION AND CYSTOSCOPY

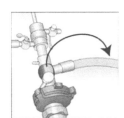

Sari Kives, M.D.
Resad P. Pasic, M.D., Ph.D.

Diagnostic hysteroscopy is ideal for assessing the uterine cavity in women with a history of abnormal bleeding, a misplaced intrauterine device, infertility, or an abnormal ultrasound. It enables direct visualization of the uterine cavity so that pathology can be identified, biopsies can be performed and small lesions can be removed.

To perform a diagnostic hysteroscopy successfully several requirements must be fulfilled.

PATIENT PREPARATION

Patients can be scheduled for diagnostic hysteroscopy after obtaining a comprehensive patient history, performing a physical examination, discussing choice of anesthesia, and obtaining informed consent. The patient is placed in dorsolithotomy position. A pelvic examination is performed to determine the size and position of the uterus. A weighted speculum in addition to a single toothed tenaculum is used to grasp the anterior lip of the cervix applying traction in order to straighten the uterine axes (Figure 1). Excessive dilatation of the cervical canal should be avoided to minimize fluid loss.

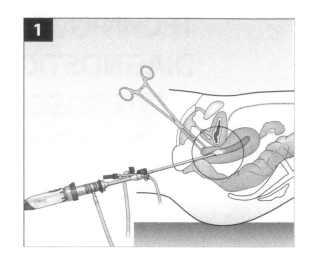

The cervical canal should be dilated equivalent to the diameter of the hysteroscopic sheath used. Sounding of the uterine cavity should be avoided since it may create lacerations of the hyperplasic endometrium which may be mistaken for intrauterine pathology. When performing a diagnostic hysteroscopy, the early proliferative stage of the menstrual cycle (day 4 to 11) is preferred as interpretation is easiest when the endometrium is the thinnest (Figure 2). Hysteroscopy performed later may be hampered by the lush, thick secretory endometrium and cause more false reports of polyps or hyperplasia (Figure 3). Endometrial biopsy or D&C should be performed after hysteroscopic examination.

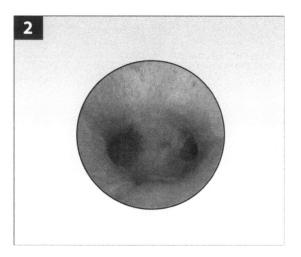

Contraindications for hysteroscopy are a recent history of pelvic inflammatory disease (PID), acute cervico-vaginal infection, and intrauterine pregnancy.

MEDIA

The uterine cavity is a potential space that may be visualized only after adequate distension. The choice of media is often arbitrary. All media should distend the uterus adequately to provide a clear and unobstructed view. The ideal media is one that does not mix easily with

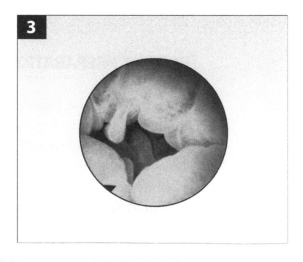

blood, does not interfere with the therapeutic procedure, and maintains a sustained intrauterine pressure to minimize bleeding and maximize visualization.

The two media most frequently used for diagnostic purposes are carbon dioxide and normal saline.

PROCEDURAL CASCADE

- BIMANUAL EXAM
- DISTENSION MEDIA CONNECTED TO INFLOW PORT
- INFLOW IS PURGED WITH LIQUID DISTENSION MEDIUM
- CERVIX ON TRACTION
- ENDOCERVIX ENGAGED WITH HYSTEROSCOPE
- CAMERA IN UPRIGHT POSITION
- BLACK HOLE FOLLOWED
- UTERINE CAVITY ENTERED AND INSPECTED
- LIGHT POST ROTATED TO VISUALIZE OSTIA
- FLOW INCREASED IF NEEDED
- ENDOCERVIX ASSESSED ON WITHDRAWAL
- HYSTEROSCOPE REMOVED
- CERVIX EXAMINED FOR BLEEDING

CARBON DIOXIDE

This media is frequently used in the outpatient setting when performing diagnostic hysteroscopy. It is quick, clean and simple and allows excellent visualization. It does not require any monitoring of fluid status. The CO_2 gas is delivered via an insufflator that limits the flow rate to a maximum of 100 mL/min and the pressure to a maximum of 200 mm Hg, although the insufflation pressure should never exceed 100 mmHg. As the gas is pumped into the uterine cavity, annoying bubbles may form but these usually disappear within a few minutes. To help clear the bubbles the insufflation pressure should be lowered and the scope can be inserted all the way to the fundus and then slowly withdrawn toward the cervical ostium.

NORMAL SALINE

Saline is readily available, inexpensive, and easy to use. The solution passes easily through the fallopian tubes and is absorbed by the peritoneal cavity. Normal saline cannot be used if electrosurgery with the traditional resectoscope is contemplated. Switching from normal saline to a non-conducting media is, however, an acceptable option if electrosurgery is needed. Alternatively, the VersaPoint™ system (Gynecare, Inc) uses normal saline as its primary media, reducing the risk of electrolyte imbalances with resection. If large volumes of saline enter the circulation, fluid overload can still occur and therefore the amount of fluid should still be monitored.

Liquid media less frequently used for diagnostic purposes include Hyskon, Glycine, and Sorbitol. All media are discussed in detail in Chapter 3.

DELIVERY SYSTEM FOR MEDIA

The use of carbon dioxide requires an insufflator that limits the rate of flow (Figure 4). In patients with patent fallopian tubes the flow rate is between 30 to 40 mL/min and the average intrauterine pressure is 60 to 80 mmHg. This insufflator operates at high pressures and low volumes in contrast to the laparoscopic insufflator, which relies on low pressure and high volumes. Laparoscopic insufflators cannot be used for hysteroscopy. Before inserting the hysteroscope the tubing should be flushed with CO_2 to eliminate air and minimize the chance of gas embolism. The Trendelenburg position should also be avoided with hysteroscopy because of the increased potential risk of gas embolism. Over distension may create a "negative" hysteroscopic appearance when using CO_2 as the distension media. Slowly deflating the uterine cavity and reinspecting the endometrial surfaces for fibroids or polyps will result in more accurate findings.

Normal saline is used most frequently for diagnostic purposes and does not require a special delivery system. Low viscosity media also do not require a special delivery system when used for diagnostic purposes.

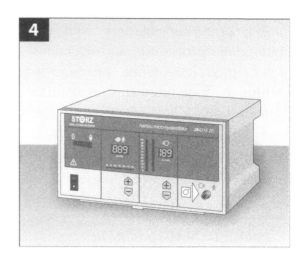

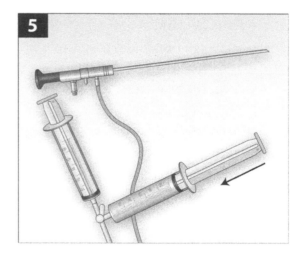

The simplest delivery system is a 60 cc syringe attached to IV tubing and then to the hysteroscope (Figure 5). This method allows a quick and easy approach to visualizing the uterine cavity and deciding on whether a further operative treatment is needed. This method is limited to diagnostic purposes only and it is exclusively used with a one channel 5 mm hysteroscopic sheath. In this technique, the intrauterine pressure may rise up to 200 mmHg to achieve adequate visualization but as minimal fluid (< 60cc) is required, this procedure is considered very safe. This delivery system requires an assistant to instill the fluid while the operator is performing the procedure.

Normal saline can also be instilled by connecting an IV bag to the hysteroscope with IV tubing (Figure 6). This system relies solely on gravity. To attain adequate visualization the IV bag must be no more and no less then 100 cm above the uterus to achieve an intrauterine pressure no greater then 75 mmHg. A blood pressure cuff can be placed around the IV bag and insufflated to 80 to 120 mm Hg to increase the flow and ensure consistent distension of the uterine cavity. The fluid output must be calculated manually but the fluid required is rarely greater than 1 liter.

If gravity is not sufficient to provide adequate visualization of the uterine cavity, or if an operative procedure is to be performed, hysteroscopy pumps are utilized (Figure 7). Hysteroscopy pumps are combined irrigation and suction devices which allow intrauterine pressure to be set and regulated. They allow controlled and precise irrigation and distention of the uterine cavity by connecting to the inflow and the outflow valve of the hysteroscopy sheath.

Specialty fluid management systems are designed to accurately measure all inputs and outputs of fluids used. These systems are used frequently when performing operative hysteroscopy or with

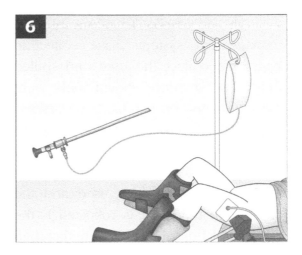

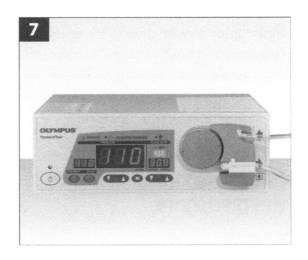

use of high viscosity liquid media. Diagnostic hysteroscopy rarely results in excessive fluid loss to warrant a more expensive fluid management system. When a diagnostic hysteroscopy is performed prior to commencing an operative procedure a fluid management system may be used. The basic principle of all fluid management systems consists of monitoring the amount of fluid used and monitoring the amount of fluid that is collected after the fluid passes through the uterus. Therefore all fluid management systems have collection bags that collect the used and spilled fluid. The operator should make sure that the collection bag has been properly placed and taped to patient's legs to avoid any spillage of fluid out of the collection bag to the floor. The difference in the amount of fluid used and the amount of fluid that is collected is the amount of fluid that has been absorbed in general circulation.

Many systems exist for monitoring input and output during hysteroscopy (Figure 8). These systems significantly reduce the major risks of operative hysteroscopy, which include fluid overload and electrolyte imbalances (See Chapter 3).

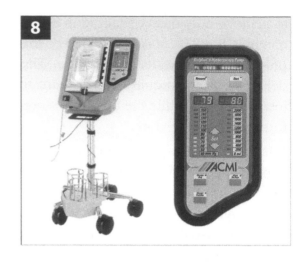

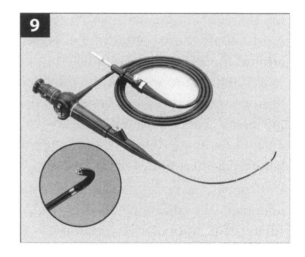

CHOOSING THE APPROPRIATE HYSTEROSCOPE

FLEXIBLE

Flexible steerable diagnostic hysteroscopes can have an even smaller diameter of 3 mm with no outer sheath and are ideal for office hysteroscopy. They are capable of being bent in many directions. The distal tip of the flexible scope can be deflected up or down 90° to 110° to view the inner ostium (Figure 9). The scope has a distal fiber optic system rather than the traditional lenses with a resulting decrease in resolution. The flexible distal end does not always pass through a stenotic or tight cervical os

with as much ease as a rigid telescope. These scopes also have a greater learning curve than the simple diagnostic sheath and telescope.

RIGID TELESCOPES

The hysteroscopes most commonly used have 12°, 25° or 30° lenses. The lens angle is engraved on the proximal part of every scope by the eye piece so the operator can distinguish between different scopes. The lens angle is offset from the scope so that rotation of the scope enlarges the field of view. A 0° lens is centered with the axis of the scope making the cornual areas difficult to visualize. The 25° lens is slanted 25° from the center in the direction opposite from the light attachment on the scope (Figure 10). This is standard for every telescope produced and it can help the operator distinguish in what direction he/she is looking. The direction is always away from the light source attachment. The 25° scope is preferred for diagnostic purposes as it allows easy observation of the uterine horns and tubal ostia when the telescope is rotated to the left or right. In order to visualize the right ostia the operator should keep the camera in upright position, hold the light cable and rotate the scope clockwise until the right ostia appears in his view field. Sometimes the scope axis should be changed by moving the camera toward the patient's left side in order to point the tip of the scope toward the right ostia (Figure 11). The 12° lens can also be used for diagnostic hysteroscopy but it may not be optimal for viewing the ostia if they are situated too far lateral. The 12° lens is usually preferred when using the resectoscope since it offers enough deviation to view the tip of the active electrode.

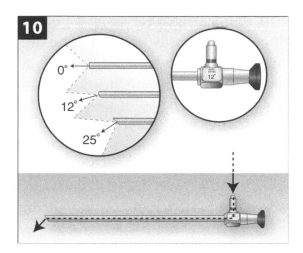

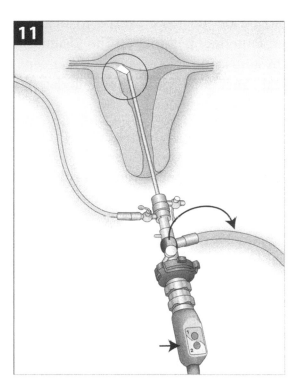

SHEATH/BRIDGE

When performing a diagnostic hysteroscopy in the office it is preferable to have a narrow sheath, as it is associated with less manipulation and discomfort. A wider range of choice in operative sheaths may be used when the patient is under general anesthesia because dilation may be performed more comfortably.

A simple diagnostic sheath 3.5 mm to 5 mm in diameter is used most frequently to perform a diagnostic hysteroscopy. This sheath has a port for instilling either liquid or gas media. No accessory port is present. The 60 cc syringe or IV bag filled with saline and connected with IV tubing to the hysteroscope is used for distention and adequate visualization of the uterine cavity. If any abnormalities are observed the operator can decide at that moment if he/she will use the operative hysteroscope or the resectoscope to treat the intrauterine pathology. The diagnostic hysteroscope is removed and the cervical canal is dilated to accommodate the chosen instrument.

A simple operative sheath 6–7 mm in diameter may also be used for diagnostic purposes, but it requires additional dilatation of the cervical canal. An operative sheath has an inflow and outflow channel for the liquid to be cleared. The distention media is delivered either from the IV bag by gravity or using a hysteroscopy pump. This sheath has stopcocks on either side for instillation of the media. The alternative side is fitted with a rubber nipple to prevent loss of media while the accessory port is being used to biopsy or remove a polyp. This system uses semi-rigid instruments for treatment of uterine pathology (Figure 12). There are also operative hysteroscopes with rigid instruments called optical forceps. The optical forceps house the scope and have scissor-like

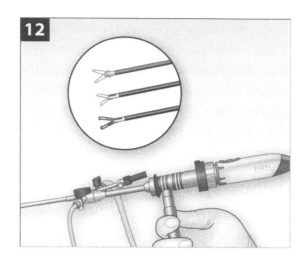

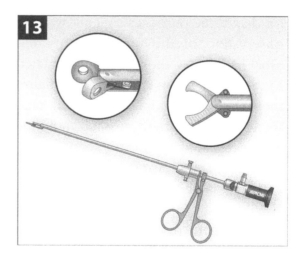

handles that operate the tip of the instrument (Figure 13). The rigid instruments are more sturdy and robust and may offer better assistance in removal of large polyps. The instrument is already part of the hysteroscope sheath and the telescope is inserted along the instrument shaft to aid in the visualization of the instrument tip. The tip of the instrument can be in the form of scissors or forceps.

The typical 9 mm diameter operative resectoscope sheath is much larger and requires dilation of the cervix (Figure 14). It has multi-channel sheaths that are isolated from each other and allow rinsing of the uterine cavity. One channel exists for the scope, one for instillation of media, and one to remove media and clear blood clot and debris without significant intrauterine variations in pressure. These hysteroscopes require a pump for fluid delivery. A 12° lens is most frequently used with the operative sheath, and different electrodes can be added for treatment of intrauterine pathology. A fluid management system is generally used with resectoscopes for distention and visualization of the uterine cavity.

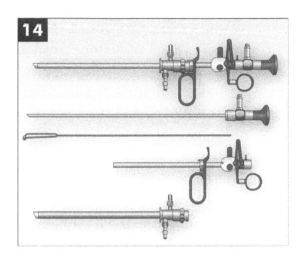

DILATION OF CERVIX

Dilation is rarely required for diagnostic hysteroscopy because the hysteroscope selected is usually ≤ 5 mm in diameter. If the cervix has to be dilated, the Pratt or Hagar dilator may be used to dilate the external and internal os. Over-dilation should be avoided, as it may result in escape of media via the cervical canal and, ultimately, poor visualization. The multiparous cervix rarely has to be dilated because of its patulous nature. A paracervical block can be performed first to provide local anesthesia. Local anesthesia is rarely needed if the hysteroscope selected is a small caliber sheath (≤ 5 mm). Occasionally, nulli-

parous or post-menopausal patients will require cervical dilation prior to hysteroscopy. Laminaria can be inserted the night before surgery. Alternatively the patient may receive 200–400 mg misoprostol vaginally 4 hours prior to the procedure. The cervical canal should be routinely examined during the insertion of the hysteroscope. Cervical adhesions, polyps, cervical atresia, and other abnormalities can easily be diagnosed.

MANEUVERING THE HYSTEROSCOPE

The hysteroscope with the attached camera is held in the operator's dominant hand. The camera should always remain fixed and in the upright position. The hysteroscope and its 5 mm sheath are advanced through the endocervical canal under direct vision and into the uterine cavity. The hysteroscope is advanced on an angle in order to offset the lens angle and to obtain a straight view of the endocervical canal (Figure 15). The pathway to the uterine cavity is outlined by a black hole, which appears following insertion of the hysteroscope. This black hole leads to the fundus of the uterus and should be visible always at the 6 o'clock position. If the passage is impaired or blocked and the black hole is lost, withdraw the hysteroscope a few millimeters and search for the cavity. Often the hysteroscope will need to be moved two steps forward and then one step back to keep this pathway in view. It is important to remember never to force the passage of the hysteroscope as this could traumatize the mucosa leading to false passage and perforation. The tenaculum on the cervix is held in the non-dominant hand to apply constant traction on the cervix. If the uterus is anteverted an attempt is made to insert the hysteroscope with the lens directed upward (Figure 15). If however the uterus is retroverted the lens should be directed downward (Figure 16). The light cord will assist the operator in determining in what position the lens is directed. The hysteroscope lens is always directed 180° away from the light cord insertion.

It is also important to be aware of the degree of the scope. Most diagnostic scopes have 25° or 30° lenses and as a result they deflect light to the area of interest at a 25° or 30° angle. Less light is directed to the surrounding area.

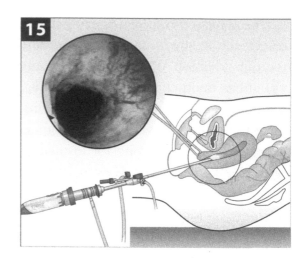

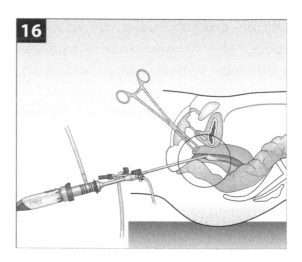

ASSESSING THE UTERUS

To clearly visualize the uterus and tubal ostia the walls of the uterus should be distended to their maximum using CO_2 or a fluid medium. A uterine pressure of 60–80 mmHg is necessary for adequate visualization. The uterine cavity should be examined systematically starting with the cavity and followed by the tubal ostia, endometrium, internal os, and cervix. Hysteroscopy should be performed ideally in the post-menstrual period to enhance visualization. In order to visualize the right ostium the operator should hold the camera in the upright position in the non-dominant hand. The light cable is held in the dominant hand and the scope is rotated clockwise until the right ostium appears in his/her view. Sometimes the scope axis can also be changed by moving the camera toward the patient's left side in order to point the tip of the scope toward the right ostium (Figure 17). The light cord acts as a guide and directs the hysteroscope to the area of interest. To visualize the left ostium, the camera should remain fixed and in the upright position, the light cable should be rotated counterclockwise, and the axis of the scope should be moved so the tip of the hysteroscope is pointing toward the left ostium (Figure 18).

TROUBLESHOOTING

FLUID LOSS

When performing hysteroscopy excessive fluid may be lost through the cervix due to either a patulous cervix or over dilation. Excessive fluid loss can result in a less then optimal view. In the event of fluid loss one can prevent leakage with a Gimpelson's tenaculum, an endoloop placed around the cervix, or two single-toothed tenacula placed side by side on the cervix (Figure 19).

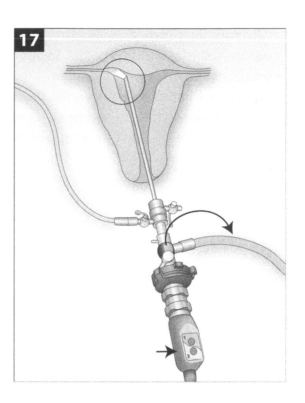

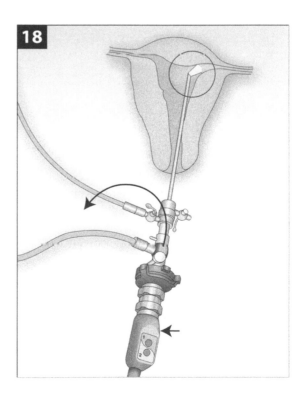

Factors that can directly affect the outflow of distension media include leakage at the cervical junction, the dimensional interface between the inner and outer sheaths of a continuous flow sheath, amount of active suction placed on the outflow tract, the use of ancillary aspiration, transtubal passage into the peritoneal cavity, and intravasation into the vascular network of the uterus.

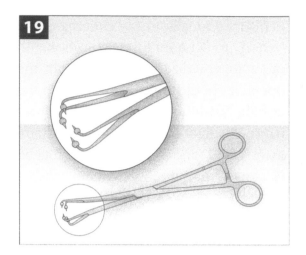

INADEQUATE UTERINE DISTENSION

- Leakage at cervix
- Equipment leakage
- Bent tubing
- Excessive outflow
- Obstruction at stopcock
- Significant intravasation
- Uterine rupture

UTERINE OUTFLOW FACTORS

- Leakage at cervix
- Continuous flow sheath interface
- Outflow suction
- Transtubal loss
- Intravasation

LOSS OF VISION

When performing diagnostic hysteroscopy, maintaining a sustained intrauterine pressure will minimize bleeding and maximize visualization. If the endoscopic view is impaired by blood or secretions adhering to the lens, pressing the lens against the uterine fundus will often restore the view. Occasionally loss of vision will occur due to fluctuations in the intrauterine pressure. In this event, closing the out valve on the multi-channel sleeve may improve the situation. The multi-channel sheath has an in-valve for instillation of media and an out-valve to remove media and clear blood clots and debris. By closing the out-valve for short periods of time, visualization may improve by creating a more stable intrauterine pressure. Caution, this should only be momentary.

COPIOUS BLEEDING

When performing a diagnostic hysteroscopy copious bleeding may occur. Irrigating with 100–300 cc of fluid, aspirating the fluid with a syringe, and then redistending will usually lead to an improved view. The resectoscope has a multi-channel sleeve which helps to remove blood clots and debris continuously. Always make sure that the out flow valve is open. The resectoscope may result in more acute bleeding. Treatments for acute bleeding include inserting an intrauterine Foley catheter or injecting a diluted pitressin solution into the cervix.

HOW TO USE THE RESECTOSCOPE

The working element is the main part of the resectoscope to which cutting loops or coagulating electrodes are attached. The sheath of the resectoscope is 9 mm in diameter and requires dilation of the cervix. It has multi-channel sheaths that are isolated from each other and allow rinsing of the uterine cavity. One channel is for instillation of media and the other to remove fluid and to clear blood clots and debris without significant intrauterine variations in pressure. A 12° lens is most frequently used with the operative sheath, and different electrodes can be added for treatment of intrauterine pathology. A fluid management system is generally used

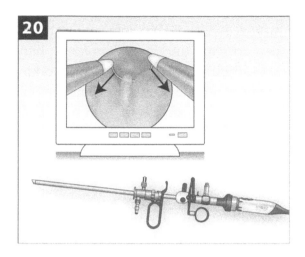

with the resectoscope for distention and visualization of the uterine cavity and to monitor the fluid loss accurately.

The resectoscope is maneuvered in the same manner as a diagnostic hysteroscope since the same principles apply to both. The camera should always remain fixed and in the upright position. After inserting the resectoscope, the light cord assists the operator in orienting the loop or the roller ball along the uterine walls. The loop or roller ball is usually directed 180° away from the light cord (Figure 20). The camera should always be held in the upright position with the non-dominant hand. When the camera is attached a loop electrode can be visualized at the tip of the hysteroscope. The loop electrode can be moved forward by squeezing the handle on the working element. The loop or rollerball should only be activated under direct vision as the electrode is being drawn toward the cervix and into the sheath. To reach the patient's left lateral uterine wall, the camera in the non-dominant hand should be kept steady, and the working element in the dominant hand should be rotated around its axis in a counter-clockwise direction (Figure 21). To reach the right uterine wall, the camera should be held steady in the upright position and the working element in the dominant hand should be rotated in a clockwise direction turning the loop at the tip of the hysteroscope toward the right uterine wall (Figure 22). The working element held by the dominant hand should be rotated 360° in order to reach all parts of the uterine cavity while the laparoscopic camera is held steady in the upright position by the non-dominant hand.

HOW TO PERFORM CYSTOSCOPY

With the advancement of laparoscopic surgery and the new approach of treating urinary stress incontinence with TVT there is an increased requirement for gynecologic surgeons to be proficient in performing cystoscopy. Cystoscopy should not be viewed differently than performing hysteroscopy. A cystoscope should be used instead of the hysteroscope, although they work on the same principle. Normal saline solution can be used for dilatation of the bladder and a laparoscopic camera should always be connected to the cystoscope to make the procedure more comfortable for the surgeon.

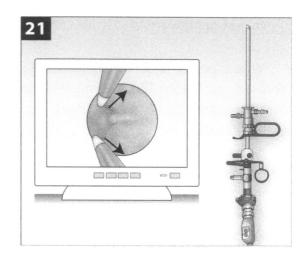

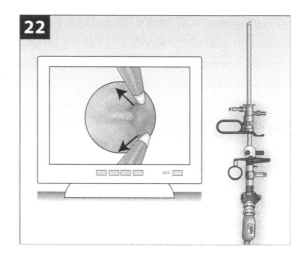

The urethra, bladder neck, and trigone of the bladder are easily inspected with the use of a 30° or 70° cystoscope using the same basic principles as diagnostic hysteroscopy. No dilation of the urethral meatus is required. The vast majority of women require no anesthesia for this procedure but in most cases cystoscopy is carried out under general anesthesia at the completion of a major gynecologic procedure. The camera should always remain fixed and in the upright position. The urethra is visualized throughout its length as the cystoscope is inserted. After inserting the cystoscope, the light cord assists in orienting the lens as the operator inspects the bladder walls, the trigone, and the ureteric orifices. The cystoscope lens is always directed 180° away from the light cord.

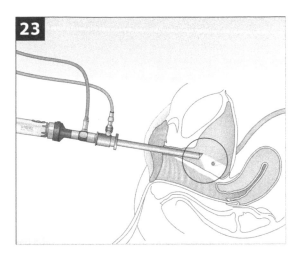

The ureteric orifices are located below the urethra and cannot be visualized with the 0° scope. The operator therefore should ideally use a 70° scope to visualize the orifices (Figure 23). In order to visualize the patient's right orifice, the camera should be raised and moved toward the patient's left leg pointing the tip of the cystoscope down toward the patient's right ureteral orifice. The camera should always be kept in the upright position. The light cord should be rotated 45° clockwise pointing the 70° lens toward the patient's right side until the right ureteral orifice is found. In order to visualize the left ureteral orifice, the camera should be held in the upright position and moved toward the patient's right leg changing the axis of the scope, and pointing the tip of the cystoscope toward the left ureteral orifice. The light cord should be rotated counterclockwise until the left ureteral orifice is visualized (Figure 24).

Indigo carmine may be administered intravenously approximately 2 to 3 minutes prior to performing a cystoscopy.

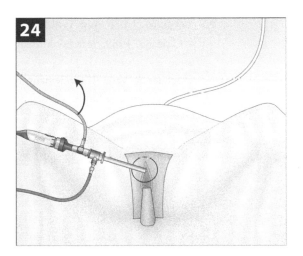

Indigo carmine allows for the clear visualization of both ureteric orifices as it causes the urine to turn blue.

After visualization of both ureteral ostia, the camera is kept steady in the upright position and the light cable is rotated downward pointing the tip of the cystoscope toward the bladder dome and the rest of the bladder is inspected.

SUGGESTED READING:

Corfman R, Diamond M, DeCherney A. Complications of Laparoscopy and Hysteroscopy, Oxford, 1993, Blackwell Scientific Publications

Baggish M, Barbot J, Valle R. Diagnostic and Operative Hysterocopy: Text and Atlas, Chicago, 1989, Year Book Medical Publishers Inc

Seigler A, Valle R, Lindemann H, Mencaglia L. Therapeutic Hysteroscopy Indications and Techniques, St Louis, 1990, The C.V. Mosby Company

OFFICE HYSTEROSCOPY

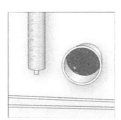

Beverly R. Love, M.D.
Roosevelt McCorvey, M.D.

Office hysteroscopy is defined as an office-based procedure performed under local anesthesia (OHULA). This pneumonic stands for OFFICE HYSTERSCOPY UNDER LOCAL ANESTHESIA. Most gynecologists perform hysteroscopy in outpatient surgery centers and hospitals. In fact only 20% of gynecologists perform hysteroscopy at all. More importantly, only 5% of gynecologists participate in office hysteroscopy. Factors that explain the low utilization of office hysteroscopy by gynecologists include lack of knowledge about this technique which is probably a reflection of lack of training in hysteroscopy in the residency program. Therefore, there is a lack of awareness about the diagnostic and therapeutic capability of hysteroscopy. The lack of training in local anesthesia for office hysteroscopy suggests a large reason for the minority of gyn participation in this technique. The fact that there is a significant money outlay for office hysteroscopy is probably the second most significant factor preventing gynecologists from involvement in this endeavor. The corollary is that reimbursement for office hysteroscopy is sorely lacking. The combination of all of these factors adds up to the lack of interest in office hysteroscopy. It

Chapter 7

84 | OFFICE HYSTEROSCOPY . . . .

is our hope that in the future these factors will change and that more gynecologists will perform office hysteroscopy.

INDICATIONS FOR OFFICE HYSTEROSCOPY

Any patient that presents with abnormal uterine bleeding could be a candidate for OHULA. The contraindications for this procedure include pregnancy, endometritis, PID, cervical cancer, fear of local anesthesia, and documented allergy to local anesthesia. The indications for abnormal bleeding may include the following diagnoses: dysfunctional uterine bleeding, menorrhagia, intramural myomas (rule out submucous myomas), infertility, (rule out intra-uterine septum), intrauterine polyps, endo-cervical polyps, postmenopausal bleeding, amenorrhea, post endometrial ablation bleeding, and other abnormal bleeding.

CHOOSING THE HOSPITAL SETTING

- APPREHENSIVE PATIENT
- NEED FOR EXTENSIVE SURGICAL PROCEDURE
- CERVICAL STENOSIS
- POTENTIAL FOR SUPPLEMENTAL LAPAROSCOPY

PATIENT SELECTION

A relative contraindication for OHULA is a stenotic cervix or suspected intrauterine adhesions. The treatment of patients with suspected intrauterine adhesions or synechia are problematic in the office setting because of the increased risk for uterine perforation. We would recommend that most cases of suspected intrauterine adhesions be treated in the surgi-center or out-patient hospital.

We show all of our OHULA patients an educational video on hysteroscopy by Milner-Fenwick. This serves the purpose of decreasing patients' fears about the procedure. Patients are required to sign informed consent for OHULA. We give the patients the risks and benefits of OHULA. Certainly, the risks of OHULA are low and the benefits are high including decreased cost to the patient and sometimes an instantaneous diagnosis with video hysteroscopy. A positive benefit to one's practice is that patients will tell their friends and family that they could see their "insides" and this may induce more patients to come to the practice.

OFFICE HYSTEROSCOPY

- MOST PATIENTS WILL REQUIRE NO ANESTHESIA
- GIVE ORAL ANALGESIC 30 TO 60 MIN BEFORE PROCEDURE
- PARACERVICAL AND INTRACERVICAL BLOCKS

PREOPERATIVE ANTIBIOTICS?

- HIGH RISK PATIENTS
- VALVULAR DISEASE
- DIABETES MELLITUS
- PRIOR PID
- HIGH DOSE CORTICOSTEROIDS

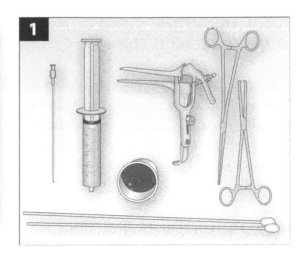

TECHNIQUE FOR OHULA

A dedicated room for office hysteroscopy is advantageous. Some of the basic equipment that you will need for the OHULA room will include:

- Exam table that will allow head elevation
- Adjustable stool
- Exam light
- Open-sided speculum
- Video camera
- Video monitor with a VCR
- Local anesthetics, syringes, small gauge needles (21 or smaller), needle extender (Figure 1)
- Hysteroscopes (flexible and/or small rigid) (Figure 2)
- Operative resectoscope (22 Fr) Storz and (24 Fr) R. Wolf
- Dilators up to a Hegar 8
- Optional, IV set-up only for operative resectoscopes or hysteroscopic endometrial ablations

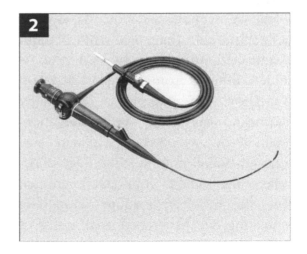

- 4 by 4 gauzes
- Set-up and sterilization solutions (Cidex)
- Cart for the video set-up
- Mayo stands for the hysteroscopes and the ancillary instruments
- Automatic fluid monitor for rollerball endometrial ablations and resections
- Any of the global endometrial ablation instruments

LOCAL ANESTHESIA
WITH INTRAVENOUS SEDATION

Local anesthesia involves simple infiltration of local anesthetic subcutaneously, submucosally, or near neurovascular bundles. A 1% Xylocaine solution is injected barely beneath the cervicovaginal mucosa at 5 o'clock and 7 o'clock position (Figure 3). Three to 4 cc of the anesthetic solution injected in each ligament is adequate for pain control.

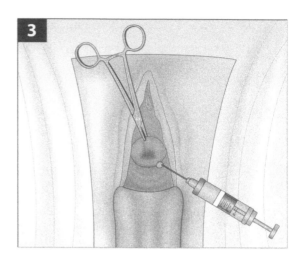

Some OHULA patients may require more than local anesthesia and need some intravenous sedation. We suggest a technique that we call Patient Controlled Anesthesia or PCA. PCA is much different from Conscious Sedation whereby the patient is essentially "knocked out" with the IV sedation. With PCA, we give the patient just enough sedation to take the edge off or make the patient comfortable enough for the brief procedure. Generally speaking, we have used small doses of Fentanyl ranging from 25 mcg to 100 mcg depending on the size of the patient. Another component of our PCA technique involves VOLONELGESIA and VIDEOGESIA. VOLONELGESIA refers to the use of vocal stimuli or talking to the patient while you perform OHULA. VIDEOGESIA is the use of the video monitor whereby the patient can be distracted by the images of her "insides". The most important aspect of PCA is that the hysteroscopist must become comfortable with the idea of talking with the patient while procedures are being conducted. The PCA procedures will be more successful if the hysteroscopist participates with VOLONELGESIA. We recommend that the hysteroscopist be proctored or work with an office based hysteroscopist to make these procedures more successful.

PROCEDURE

First, the patient must have a complete history and physical. Then OHULA must be explained to the patient by the clinician both verbally and preferably with a patient video. The patient must understand that the procedure will be performed under local anesthesia and that the recovery time in the office will be brief. The patient is required to sign a consent form.

We use the following steps for OHULA:

• After the patient is dressed with the office gown, pre-medication is given with Atropine 0.4mg and Toradal 30mg.

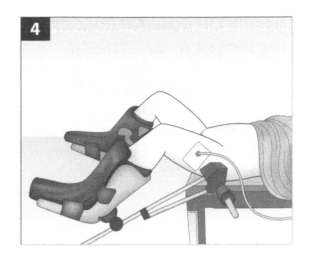

- Atropine may reduce the vasovagal reactions and Toradal may reduce uterine cramping secondary to antiprostaglandin activity.

- The patient is escorted to the OHULA room.

- Next, the patient is placed on the OHULA table in the Allen stirrups or knee stirrups (Figure 4).

- The open-sided speculum is inserted into the vagina.

- The cervix is prepped with Betadine.

- Hurricane Spray is applied to the cervix, then wait a few minutes.

- 10 cc of 1% Xylocaine is used for a paracervical block.

- A tenaculum may be used to hold the cervix while the flexible hysteroscope is inserted under video direction (Figure 5).

- If a rigid hysteroscope is used, the cervix may require some dilation prior to insertion.

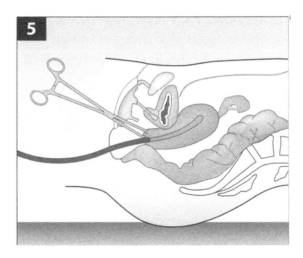

- The insufflation media may be CO_2 or fluid by IV hanging bag normal saline or syringe (50 cc).

- Then the cavity may be inspected noting the anatomical markers (the tubal ostia) working down to the endocervix.

- We use a 25-inch monitor so the patient can see what we see. If we note pathology, it is immediately addressed to the patient.

- After the scope is removed, an endometrial aspirate biopsy is obtained.

- Then all instruments are removed from the patient. The patient is cleaned up, allowed to dress, and may leave the office shortly.

- A follow-up appointment is made for 2 weeks to discuss the findings and the endometrial biopsy results.

OFFICE MICROHYSTEROSCOPY UNDER LOCAL ANESTHESIA

Most of our OHULAs have been performed with the 4 mm hysteroscope from the Richard Wolf Company (Figure 6). Occasionally, we have encountered difficulty with the patient who has a stenotic cervix necessitating the use of a flexible microhysteroscope from Leisengang. With the flexible hysteroscope, the dilating agent, either CO_2 gas or normal saline, will open up the cervix. An adequate diagnostic hysteroscopy can be performed but the image is smaller on the video monitor. Additional experience with the rigid scope is needed before becoming comfortable with the flexible hysteroscope.

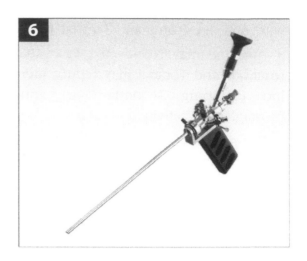

6

DOCUMENTATION

- DESCRIPTIVE
- ANATOMICAL DRAWINGS
- DIGITAL PHOTOGRAPHY
- VIDEO

RISKS WITH OHULA

There are very few risks associated with the OHULA procedure. The main long-term risk is intrauterine infection. These particular infections are extremely rare. The only intra-operative risks that one must ponder are vasovagal reaction, intravascular injection of local anesthetics, and uterine perforation. With the pre-operative use of Atropine, the majority of vasovagal reactions are eliminated. The intravascular injection problem can be abated by careful technique and always aspirating before injecting local anesthetics. If perforation occurs during OHULA, the procedure must be terminated. Then treat the patient with observation and post-operative antibiotics.

ADVANTAGES OF OHULA

The OHULA procedure has several advantages over conventional hospital or surgery center hysteroscopy including convenience for the patient and the physician, a less costly procedure, instantaneous diagnosis in some cases, some reassurance for patients with post-menopausal bleeding, increased physician reimbursement, and positive promotion for the physician's practice.

OFFICE HYSTEROSCOPY BENEFITS

- CONSCIOUS PATIENT INTEGRATION
- MINIMAL TO NO ANESTHESIA
- NO CONCERN FOR OPERATING ROOM SCHEDULE
- SHORT PROCEDURE TIME
- POTENTIAL FOR SIMULTANEOUS DIAGNOSIS AND TREATMENT
- REDUCED DIRECT AND INDIRECT COSTS

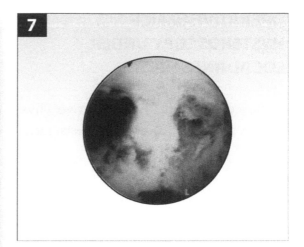

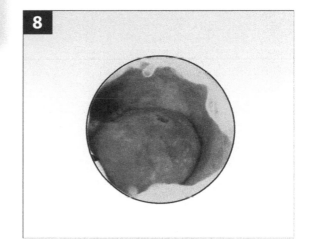

EXPERIENCE WITH OHULA

In our 20 years performing OHULA, we have identified a number of pathologies in our facility, including endometrial hyperplasia, atrophic endometrium, endometrial septa (Figure 7), endometrial polyps (Figure 8), Asherman's syndrome, submucous myomas (Figure 9) and early endometrial cancer. The majority of our patients have been satisfied with the procedure and we have had no significant complications in our OHULA practice. We believe that patients have a better appreciation for their problems when they have the ability to allow them to see inside the uterus in the office setting.

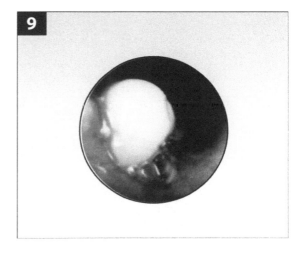

Chapter 7

90 | OFFICE HYSTEROSCOPY . . . .

OPERATIVE OFFICE HYSTEROSCOPY UNDER LOCAL ANESTHESIA

Procedures using operative hysteroscopy under local anesthesia range from rollerball endometrial ablations, ablations of submucous myomas, and global hysteroscopic endometrial ablations. These procedures will be described in detail in Chapters 14–18.

SUGGESTED READING:

Isaacson K. Office Hysteroscopy, Mosby Year Book, 1966

McCorvey R, Love B, Office HTA under local anesthesia,
Alternatives to hysterectomy. Proceedings from the World Congress on Alternatives
to Hysterectomy, Miami, Fla., AAGL 2000, p. 19

Bettochi S, et al. What does diagnostic hysteroscopy mean today? Curr Opinion.
Obstet Gynecol 2003; Aug 15(4):303-8 Review

HYSTEROSCOPY FOR INFERTILITY

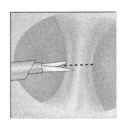

Andrew L. de Fazio, M.D.
Ceana Nezhat, M.D.

INTRODUCTION

Infertility is a common problem in today's society affecting about 15% of couples. There are multiple etiologies, with the most common being male factor (35%) and female tubal/pelvic factor (35%). Anovulation is the cause in 15% of cases and approximately 10–15% of infertility is unexplained. Congenital uterine anomalies are present in about 0.1% to 0.5% of the population and 20% of females with these anomalies experience reproductive failures, usually in the form of recurrent spontaneous abortions and preterm delivery. These anomalies result from abnormalities in lateral fusion of the mullerian ducts and include defects such as uterus didelphys, unicornuate and bicornuate uterus, and septate uterus (Figure 1). The septate uterus is the most common of these anomalies and is associated with the highest risk of pregnancy loss. It is also unique among these anomalies in that operative hysteroscopic correction is possible and very successful. Arcuate uterus is a variant of normal and is not associated with increased rates of infertility or pregnancy wastage. Other intrauterine

Chapter 8

94 | HYSTEROSCOPY FOR INFERTILITY ....

anatomic abnormalities such as intrauterine adhesions (Asherman's syndrome), submucous myomas and endometrial polyps are also associated with increased rates of infertility and are amenable to hysteroscopic correction. There are numerous studies reporting increased pregnancy rates in the range of 40%-80% following hysteroscopic correction of intrauterine defects although no randomized controlled trials exist. However, the results from retrospective studies are promising.

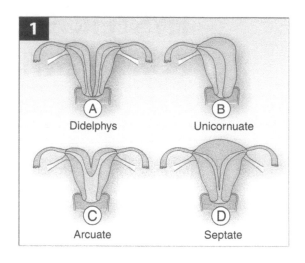

WORK-UP

Infertile patients and those with recurrent pregnancy loss must receive a thorough diagnostic evaluation. Male factor, anovulation, luteal phase defects, infectious etiologies, endocrinopathies, autoimmune disorders, and antiphospholipid syndrome must be excluded. Anatomic abnormalities must also be evaluated. Modalities such as hysterosalpingography (HSG), transvaginal ultrasonography (TVS), sonohysterography (SHG), and office hysteroscopy can be utilized. As 15% of patients with uterine anomalies can have associated urinary tract malformations, evaluation with an IVP or MRI should be considered if these anomalies are discovered.

HSG is the most commonly employed modality in evaluating the uterine cavity in the infertile patient. It provides valuable information regarding the uterine cavity but also evaluates for possible tubal pathology. However when compared to operative hysteroscopy, HSG has been found to have fairly high false positive and false negative rates in the detection of uterine pathology. Office diagnostic hysteroscopy is now being widely used for uterine cavity evaluation. A recent prospective, randomized, investigator-blinded study was performed by Brown et al. comparing the diagnostic accuracy of HSG, SHG, and outpatient hysteroscopy for evaluation of the uterine cavity in infertile women. They found no difference in the diagnostic accuracy of these modalities when used alone or in concert. Further studies need to be performed in this area.

Surgical therapy should not be employed when an incidental uterine anomaly or lesion is discovered in the absence of a history of infertility or pregnancy wastage. There is no evidence to suggest that surgical correction of uterine defects is beneficial in the setting of untried fertility. In appropriate situations, however, hysteroscopic correction of uterine defects is very successful, more cost effective, and associated with decreased morbidity when compared to previous procedures which required laparotomy. Pelvic adhesions, another contributing factor to infertility, are avoided, as is the need for cesarean section in subsequent pregnancies, and the procedure is performed in an outpatient setting.

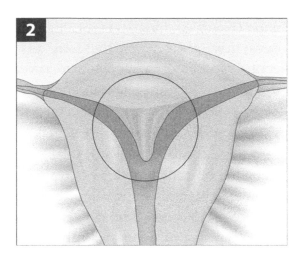

GENERAL INTRAOPERATIVE PRECAUTIONS

Operative hysteroscopy should be performed both judiciously and expeditiously. Concomitant laparoscopy may be used when appropriate such as in the treatment of uterine septa and severe intrauterine adhesions in order to avoid uterine perforation. Strict measurement of inflow and outflow of fluids must always be maintained, especially when non-electrolyte fluids are used, to avoid fluid overload and electrolyte imbalances.

UTERINE DEFECTS

SEPTATE UTERUS

As stated previously, septate uterus, the most common congenital uterine anomaly, is associated with the highest rate of pregnancy wastage and is the only congenital anomaly amenable to

hysteroscopic revision. It is thought to arise from incomplete canalization after mullerian duct fusion. It is believed to cause infertility and pregnancy wastage due to its poor vascularity and highly fibrous nature, impeding embryo implantation and subsequent normal placental growth. Septa are variable in length and usually widen as they approach the uterine fundus (Figure 2).

Septum resection via operative hysteroscopy should be scheduled for the early follicular phase or after endometrial suppression with OCP, progestins, etc., when the endometrium provides the best visualization and the risk of pregnancy is minimal. Correlation should be made with a preoperative HSG in order to ascertain the length and thickness of the septum. Concomitant laparoscopy should be performed in order to differentiate between the bicornuate uterus, which cannot be corrected hysteroscopically, and a septate uterus, and as an aid to prevent uterine perfor-

Chapter 8

96 | HYSTEROSCOPY FOR INFERTILITY . . . .

ation (Figure 3). Intraoperative IV antibiotics may be given in the form of a cephalosporin or tetracycline followed by three to four days of oral antibiotics to prevent uterine or tubal infection.

Four methods can be employed for septum resection. Hysteroscopic scissors using the operative hysteroscope are the most commonly employed instrument (Figure 4). Since the septa are usually avascular, the scissors may be used without an energy source with little to no resultant bleeding. Since no unipolar energy is needed, a safe isotonic electrolyte fluid may be used as the distention medium. The septum is transected at its midpoint, the most avascular section, proceeding from side to side until uniform transillumination is seen laparoscopically. This implies complete resection of the septum. Bleeding during resection is another sign of completion as the vascular myometrium adjacent to the septum is encountered. A uniform appearing uterine cavity visualized via a panoramic hysteroscopic view is yet another clue of complete septum resection but should not be used exclusively as a sign of procedure completion.

The resectoscope utilizing the thin electrosurgery knife may also be in septum resection (Figure 5). The same side to side cutting technique is employed using a 90–100 W cutting current and 30 W coagulating current. Since current is being employed, only non-electrolyte solutions can be used as distention media. Extra vigilance must be used

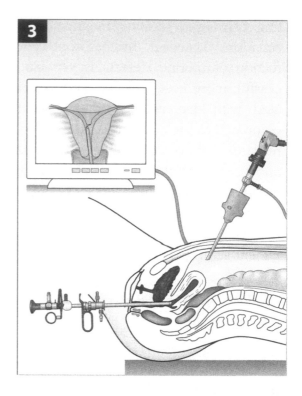

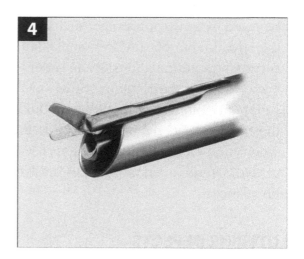

when nearing the end of the resection because one of the landmarks of complete septum resection, namely the bleeding myometrium, may be lost when the resectoscope is utilized. Lasers such as the Nd:YAG laser, or the coaxial bipolar electrode using a 200 W current, may also be utilized in a similar fashion and may be used with electrolyte solutions, as they are not conductive. Extreme care must be employed when these modalities are utilized for septum resection as they depend on heat transfer to accomplish dissection and may damage the nearby healthy endometrium. When the procedure is complete, the intrauterine pressure should be decreased to less than 60 mmHg so as not to mask bleeding vessels, which may then be selectively cauterized. An intrauterine balloon catheter may also be placed to apply direct pressure to the bleeding areas (Figure 6).

Postoperatively different modalities have been used to ensure optimal treatment. Daily oral estrogen, with or without progesterone, can be given for three to four weeks to promote endometrial growth. In addition, intrauterine devices such as balloon catheters or plastic IUDs have been placed in order to avoid apposition of the uterine walls. Although these practices are widespread, there is no data to support their usage. An HSG is usually obtained between 1 and 3 months postoperatively in order to assess the symmetry of the uterine cavity and to compare it to the preoperative study. Patients may attempt to become pregnant soon after this procedure in contrast to the long recovery period following the older open procedures.

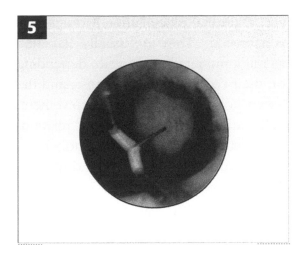

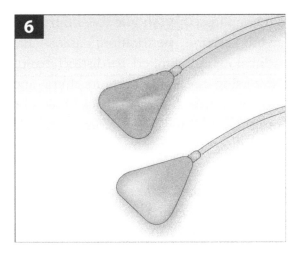

INTRAUTERINE ADHESIONS (ASHERMAN'S SYNDROME)

Asherman's syndrome describes the development of intrauterine adhesions following infection or uterine curettage for postpartum hemorrhage or incomplete or missed abortion, with subsequent damage to the basalis endometrium. These adhesions can cause infertility, recurrent pregnancy loss, or ectopic pregnancy, fetal demise, preterm labor,

Chapter 8

98 | HYSTEROSCOPY FOR INFERTILITY . . . .

and abnormal placentation if pregnancy is achieved. They are usually classified as mild, moderate, or severe, depending on their composition, thickness, and the extent of uterine cavity involvement. Valle and Sciarra studied the relationship between the severity of adhesions and pregnancy rates and found the two to be inversely related.

Preoperatively, an HSG should be obtained to ascertain the extent of the adhesions. Intraoperatively, as in the treatment of a uterine septum, concomitant laparoscopy should be utilized to avoid uterine perforation, unless the adhesions are limited to distinct bands traversing the endometrium. Intra and postoperative antibiotics should also be employed in the form of a cephalosporin or tetracycline to avoid infection.

Thin or filmy adhesions can often be lysed by dilation of the cervix. This can also be accomplished under direct visualization by pushing in the hysteroscopic sheath. Polyp forceps may also be utilized by simply opening and closing them in the endometrial cavity (Figure 7). More substantial adhesions will require division by sharp instrumentation. The same modalities employed in the resection of uterine septa may be utilized in the division of intrauterine adhesions. The hysteroscopic semirigid scissors are the instrument of choice as they do not employ a current, thereby reducing the risk of damage to the surrounding endometrium. Areas of

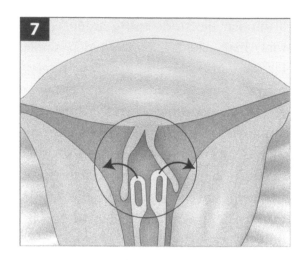

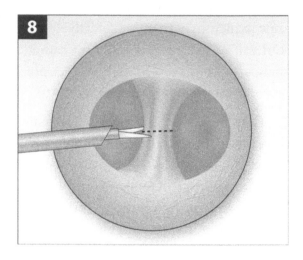

healthy endometrium are often scant in Asherman's syndrome, and it is essential to maintain their integrity so that regrowth of the endometrium is possible postoperatively. Adhesions are divided at their midpoint allowing the cut edges to retract (Figure 8). Occasionally thick stumps are left behind and require complete resection. In situations where the adhesions completely obliterate the uterine cavity, selective dissection should begin at the internal os creating a neocavity, then proceeding towards the fundus and tubal ostia, and assuring their patency. The uterine contour must be followed closely during dissection in order to avoid uterine perforation.

Postoperatively, a one-month course of estrogen is given to hyperstimulate growth of the endometrial lining. Balloon catheters or plastic IUD's can be used in cases of severe adhesions and oral antibiotics are usually continued for five to seven days postoperatively. An HSG is obtained at the completion of hormonal therapy to assess the uterine cavity and decide upon the course of care.

SUBMUCOUS MYOMAS

Submucous myomas are also associated with infertility. They can compromise the architecture and vascularity of the uterine cavity, affecting implantation, and subsequently can cause fetal wastage and malpresentation. These myomas may be either pedunculated (attached by a stalk) (Figure 9) or sessile (broad based attachment) and both types are amenable to hysteroscopic resection although different techniques are used.

Preoperatively, these patients should be evaluated with an HSG and/or a sonohysterogram to assess cavity impingement and intramuscular involvement. The procedure should once again be performed in the early follicular phase when optimal visualization is

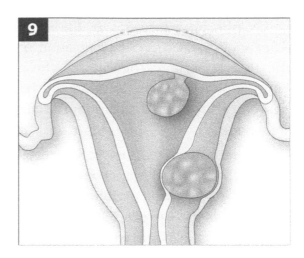

achieved. If myomas are thought to be greater than 3 cm in size, preoperative GnRH analog therapy can be employed to achieve a decrease in myoma size and vascularity, and to improve the patient's hematologic status. Maximum effect is achieved at three months. Intrauterine vasopressin may also be used to decrease intraoperative myoma vascularity. Preoperative antibiotics are used by some but are not necessary.

A variety of instruments can be used for hysteroscopic myomectomies. The resectoscope with wire loop, roller ball or roller cylinder, Nd:YAG laser, coaxial bipolar electrode, hysteroscopic scissors, and vaporizing electrodes have all been utilized. In addition, removal of pedunculated myomas can be achieved with polyp forceps if small or by the usage of polyp or unipolar snares. As always, the appropriate distention media should be used. When pedunculated myomas are substantial in size, one must assure that they are small enough to be removed through the cervix prior to transection of the stalk. After stalk transection, fragmentation of the fibroid becomes difficult, so these large pedunculated myomas should be shaved down or vaporized prior to stalk transection.

Sessile myomas are best removed by the resectoscope with a 90-degree loop utilizing the shaving technique and a cutting current between 70 W and 120 W (Figure 10). The myomas are shaved to the level of the adjacent endometrium. The cut portions of myoma are then removed, allowing the uterus to contract, causing the intramural portion of the myoma to be extruded into the cavity. By repeating this procedure, most, if not all, of the myoma may be removed hysteroscopically. If multiple myomas are present, some advocate that myomas closer to the cervical os and those located anteriorly, where air bubbles accumulate, be removed first in order to improve visualization. When fundal myomas are present, a 180° loop may be used as opposed to the usual 90° loop. Bleeding may be controlled with the roller ball or cylinder (Figure 11) or by tamponade with an intrauterine 30 cc Foley balloon.

Postoperatively, no special precautions are required. Estrogen therapy can be considered if more than one myoma is removed and two raw surfaces are in apposition. No prospective randomized trials exist regarding hysteroscopic myomectomy and subsequent fertility. A retrospective study by Bernard, et al.

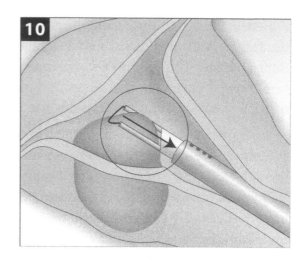

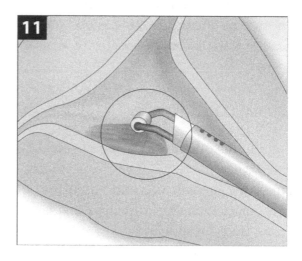

revealed that fertility after hysteroscopic myomectomy decreased if more than one myoma was removed and intramural myomas were present.

ENDOMETRIAL POLYPS

Endometrial polyps are another proposed cause of infertility and are also easily removed via hysteroscopy. Diagnostic work-up is identical to that for submucous myomas, and once again the procedure should be performed in the early follicular phase or after medical suppression to optimize visualization. Polyp forceps may be utilized as well as snare devices and hysteroscopic scissors (Figure 12). The resectoscope may also be used with the wire loop attachment (Figure 13), and multiple passes with the wire loop can remove polyps under direct visualization with or without the use of energy. Postoperatively no special precautions are required.

TUBAL DISEASE

Tubal disease is the cause of 25–30% of female infertility and approximately 20% of tubal disease is due to proximal fallopian tube obstruction. HSG is the best preoperative test for evaluation of tubal patency. When hysteroscopy is done for an infertility evaluation, the tubal ostia should be evaluated. Newer techniques are now available to treat proximal tube occlusion such as hysteroscopically assisted tubal cannulation and direct visualization with falloposcopy. Tubal cannulation is usually performed with concomitant laparoscopy. Rimbach et al. performed a multicenter prospective trial evaluating tubal

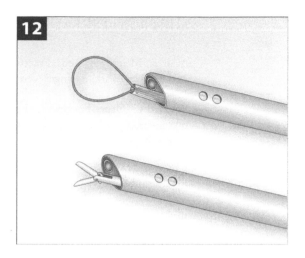

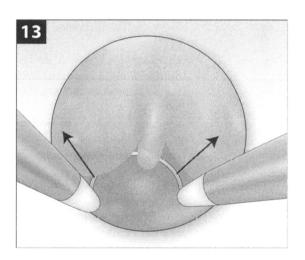

cannulation and falloposcopy and found that the procedure was successful in 69.6% of fallopian tubes. Further studies of fertility following these procedures must be performed. Refer to Chapter 10 for tubal cannulation techniques.

SUGGESTED READING:

Azziz R, Murphy AA, eds. Practical manual of operative laparoscopy and hysteroscopy, 2nd ed. New York: Springer-Verlag, 1997:286-300, 313-336

Bernard G, Darai, Poncelet C, Benifla JL, Madelenat P. Fertility after hysteroscopic myomectomy: effect of intramural myomas associated. European Journal of Obstetrics, Gynecology, & Reproductive Biology 2000;88(1):85-90

Bieber EJ, Loffer FD, eds. Gynecologic Resectoscopy. Cambridge, Massachusetts: Blackwell Science, Inc,1995

Brown SE, Coddington CC, Schnorr J, Toner JP, Gibbons W, Oehninger S. Evaluation of outpatient hysteroscopy, saline infusion hysterosonography, and hysterosalpingography in infertile women: a prospective randomized study. Fertil Steril 2000;74(5):1029-34

Donnez J, Nisolle M. An atlas of operative laparoscopy and hysteroscopy, 2nd ed. New York: The Parthenon Publishing Group Inc, 2001:449-56, 483-95

Fernandez H, Gervaise A, de Tayrac R. Operative hysteroscopy for infertility using normal saline solution and a coaxial bipolar electrode: a pilot study. Human Reproduction 2000;15(8):1773-5

Grimbizis GF, Camus M, Tarlatzis BC, Bontis JN, Devroey P. Clinical implications of uterine malformations and hysteroscopic treatment results. Human Reproduction Update 2001;7(1):161-74

Nawroth F, Schmidt T, Freise C, Foth D, Romer T. Is it possible to recommend an "optimal" postoperative management after hysteroscopic metroplasty? A retrospective study with 52 infertile patients showing a septate uterus. Acta Obstetricia et Gynecologica Scandinavica 2002;81(1):55-7

Rimbach S, Bastert G, Wallwiener D. Technical results of falloposcopy for infertility diagnosis in a large multicentre study. Human Reproduction 2001;16(5):925-30

Rock JA, Schlaff WD. The obstetric consequences of uterovaginal anomalies. Fertil Steril 1985;43:681-92

Speroff L, Glass RH, Kase NG. Clinical Gynecologic Endocrinology and Infertility, 6th ed. Baltimore, Maryland: Lippincott Williams & Wilkins, 1999:1013-56

Tulandi T, ed. Atlas of Laparoscopic and Hysteroscopic Techniques for Gynecologists, 2nd ed. London: WB Saunders, 1999:221-30, 239-54

Zabak K, Benifla JL, Uzan S. Septate uterus and reproduction disorders: current results of hysteroscopic septoplasty. Gynecologie, Obstetrique & Fertilite 2001;29(11):829-40

Zacur HA, Goodman SB. Repeated pregnancy loss. In: Wallach EE, Zacur HA, eds. Reproductive Medicine and Surgery. St. Louis: Mosby, 1995:881-94

ENDOSCOPIC TREATMENT OF UTERINE ANOMALIES

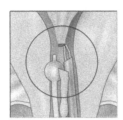

Rafael F. Valle, M.D.

The septate uterus is a uterine anomaly that frequently interferes with normal reproduction. The bicornuate uterus does not occur as frequently but may also cause pregnancy wastage and fetal malpresentations resulting in premature deliveries. The traditional methods for treatment were by classic abdominal metroplasty requiring a laparotomy and a hysterotomy. Presently, when surgical treatment of these anomalies is required, it can be provided transcervically via the hysteroscope using a variety of methods. These include hysteroscopic scissors, thermal energies via the resectoscope or hysteroscope, and laser energy via fiber optic lasers.

HYSTEROSCOPIC TECHNIQUES FOR TREATING THE SEPTATE UTERUS

PREOPERATIVE PREPARATION:

While medical preparation to thin the endometrium prior to hysteroscopic treatment of the uterine septum may be used, it is not nec-

Chapter 9

104 | ENDOSCOPIC TREATMENT OF UTERINE ANOMALIES ....

essary. When operating in the follicular phase the endometrium is thin and does not interfere with good visualization.

The instrumentation should be prepared before initiating the procedure:

• The hysteroscope/resectoscope should be properly assembled with cables for light, energy, and cameras. Bubbles should be purged from the tube delivering the distending medium.

• White balance, zooming, and focusing of the cameras should be performed.

• Check for proper patient's grounding, should electrical energy be required.

• Proper running of video taping confirmed.

• Adequate paper should be available for printing digital pictures for still photography.

• Once the procedure begins, adaptations may be necessary.

HYSTEROSCOPIC TREATMENT OF THE UTERINE SEPTUM WITH SCISSORS

The patient is placed in the dorsolithotomy position with the buttocks close to the edge of the table to avoid interfering with movements of the hysteroscope or resectoscope (Figure 1). The perineal area and vagina are cleansed with an antiseptic solution, usually Betadine solution, and after draping the patient appropriately, the bladder is catheterized. A bivalved

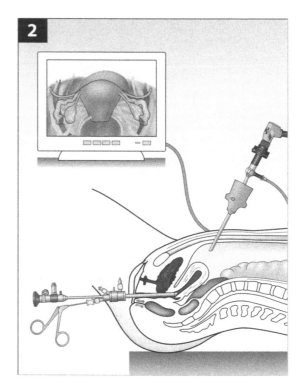

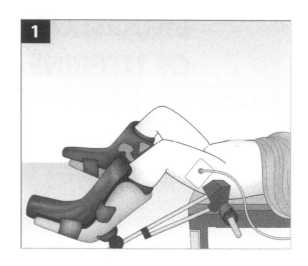

speculum with an open side is used to visualize the cervix and grasp the anterior lip of the cervix with a tenaculum. Then the bivalve speculum is replaced with a Simms retractor placed posteriorly to facilitate the cervical access of the endoscope. The cervix is gradually dilated to the size of a 7 Hegar, the hysteroscope is attached to its light source and irrigating solution and is introduced under direct vision. Blood clots and debris are washed from the cavity and the uterine septum is assessed endoscopically. A 6–8 mm outer diameter operative hysteroscope is used. Normal saline may be the most appropriate distension media for this method of treatment.

The appropriate evaluation of the uterus is done preoperatively by ultrasound to confirm the presence of a septum rather than a bicornuate uterus. Some type of monitoring method should be employed during the surgery; concomitant laparoscopy or sonography is most useful (Figure 2).

CONCOMITANT LAPAROSCOPY

When laparoscopy is used to monitor the surgery, the laparoscope is placed first, before any cervical manipulation. Usually, a 5 mm laparoscope is placed in the umbilical region and a probe in one of the lower quadrants in case the pelvic structures require manipulation. Slight Trendelenburg position will allow a complete view of the pelvic organs. The cervix is then dilated.

SONOGRAPHY

When ultrasound is used as a monitoring method for intraoperative treatment of a uterine septum, the abdomen

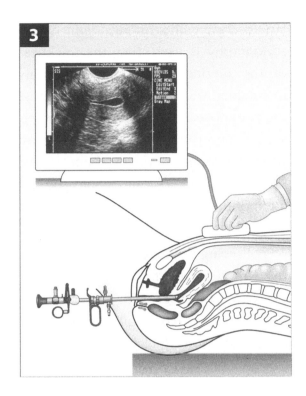

is exposed and the sonographic probe is used to determine at various planes the location of the hysteroscope and the continuous division of the septum (Figure 3).

A semi-rigid 7 Fr sharp scissors is used to divide the septum systematically from nadir to base and from side to side. Take care to maintain this division in the midline and avoid drifting towards the uterine wall to avoid unnecessary bleeding (Figure 4). From time to time, the hysteroscope is withdrawn to the internal cervical os to assess the uterine cavity's symmetry after septal division. When both uterotubal cornua are well seen and the fundal region looks symmetric, the illumination provided by the hysteroscope appears uniform by the assistant who uses

Chapter 9

106 | ENDOSCOPIC TREATMENT OF UTERINE ANOMALIES . . . .

laparoscopy with a dimmed light. When sonography is used, then the thickness of the uterine wall is also uniformly maintained. Small arteries usually cross the juxtaposed myometrium; bleeding is a good sign to stop dissection and complete the smooth convex shape of the uterine fundus. There should be no attempt to make a concave cavity as this may injure the myometrium (Figure 5).

Following the division of the septum, the intrauterine pressure is slightly decreased to observe any major arterial bleeding that may require coagulation before the procedure is completed.

The hysteroscopic division of the uterine septum with scissors is best applied to long thin septa that can easily be divided without bleeding.

ADVANTAGES TO DIVIDING A UTERINE SEPTUM WITH SCISSORS

It is an easy technique that can be performed quickly and without energy sources. The scissors can be guided under direct vision to the areas in need of treatment. Because no electricity is used, the media used to distend the uterine cavity may contain electrolytes. This provides a safety margin for utilization of fluids since more volume may be used as compared with fluids devoid of electrolytes. Rigid or semi rigid hysteroscopic scissors may be used for the excision of the septum.

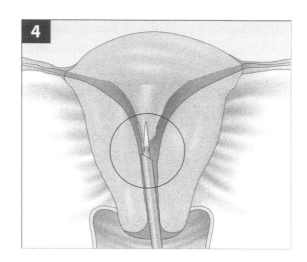

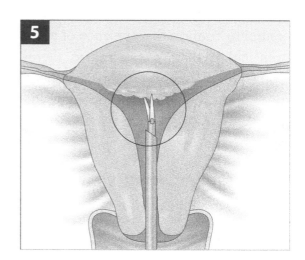

DISADVANTAGES TO USING THIS METHOD

Small scissors can become easily dulled and loose and may not cut precisely; they should be exchanged periodically and repaired. Several sets of scissors also should be at hand in case one is not functioning well. Because it is important to maintain good uterine distention and clear view of the operative field, a continuous flow hysteroscope must be used to obtain not only good distention but also a washing effect necessary for clear view.

DIVISION OF THE UTERINE SEPTUM USING THE RESECTOSCOPE

Bleeding may be encountered during the division of a thick septa or when completing the division of other septa at the base, close to the myometrium. In those cases, an 8–9 mm outer diameter gynecologic resectoscope provides an excellent washing effect of the uterine cavity to remove blood. A cutting loop is most useful and works by contact with the tissue when activating the electrode (Figure 6).

Because electrosurgery is used with the resectoscope, only fluid devoid of electrolytes can be used such as sorbitol 3%, glycine 1.3%, mannitol 5%, or glucose 5% in dextrose. One of the most commonly used distending media is glycine.

To prepare the patient, attach an appropriate return electrode plate from the electrosurgical unit to complete the electrical cycle when monopolar electrosurgery is utilized.

The uterine cervix is dilated to the size of the resectoscope used or 1–2 mm more for easier introduction and withdrawing of the resectoscope. The septum is evaluated and then divided in the middle from side to side with an electri-

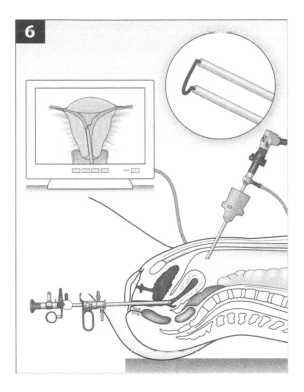

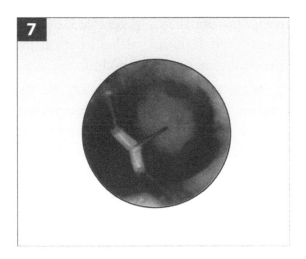

cal knife (Figure 7). The division may be completed using 100–120 W in a non-modulated (cutting) waveform. Also, a blended current of 100 W of pure cutting with 30 W of coagulating current will be useful and may be alternatively used as cutting or coagulating, should bleeding occur. The division is performed by contact of the electrode to the tissue, therefore, some forward progression is necessary taking care to proceed in a controlled, unhurried, and slow motion to prevent injury to myometrium. The operation should be monitored continuously in the same manner used when dividing the septum with scissors.

Because fluids devoid of electrolytes are used, a continuous monitoring of inflow and outflow liquids must be performed to avoid unnecessary fluid absorption. Should a fluid deficit (fluid not recovered) approach 1 liter, measure the serum sodium to determine the presence of hyponatremia and then treat appropriately. In general if there is more than 1000 mL of fluid deficit, the procedure should be aborted.

With resectoscopic division of the uterine septum, bleeding is decreased, owing to the coagulation effect of the electrical energy. The cuts are easy and the uterine cavity is washed by the continuous flow of distending fluid through the resectoscope. Some disadvantages of using of this method are: 1) the use of monopolar energy may cause injury to the myometrium and peripheral endometrium, 2) as the landmarks are lost because of the coagulating power of the electrical energy, small arterial bleeders may go unobserved unlike the use of mechanical division, 3) the necessity of using fluids devoid of electrolytes

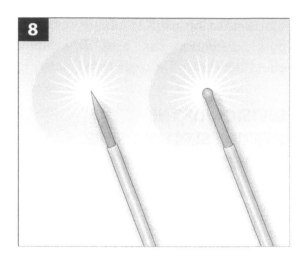

that do not permit excessive absorption (more than 1000 mL).

With the advent of the bipolar resectoscopes, the fluids may contain electrolytes, therefore giving a wider margin of safety for their utilization.

HYSTEROSCOPIC METROPLASTY WITH FIBER OPTIC LASERS

Preparation of the patient is similar to the previous method. The operative hysteroscope is used with an operating channel to manipulate the fiber optic lasers. While there are several fiber optic lasers available for this task, the Nd:YAG laser is the most commonly used with extruded or sculpted fibers as they can easily cut the tissue from side to side and complete the procedure faster than other lasers (Figure 8). Coaxial fibers with sapphire tips should not be used for this method, as these tips need to be cooled continuously either by fluid or by gases. Fluid coolant may be used, but gases should never be used in the uterus to cool the sapphire tips because of the high flow required of about 1 liter per minute. Because lasers are not conductive, electrolyte-containing fluids should be used to distend the uterine cavity. Normal saline is the most commonly used fluid for this task. A continuous flow hysteroscope also should be used, as it is important to have fluid outflow with this hysteroscopic technique to remove the debris and bubbles produced with the activated laser, and also to provide a clear view during the procedure. The usual power needed for this procedure is 20–40 W but the setting should be adapted to the laser used. Other fiber optic lasers such as the Argon and KTP-532 can also be used in this manner, although the lower power produced by these lasers makes the cutting more tedious.

Similarly, as with the other methods the division of the uterine septum should begin at the nadir of the septum in the midline dividing the septum from side to side until the base is reached (Figure 9). Care must be taken to move the fiber continuously to prevent boring into one hole. Because division of the uterine septum with fiber optic lasers may be somewhat tedious, the division should be systematic from side to side. The same precautions should be used as with division of the septum with electrocoagulation. Avoid invading the jux-

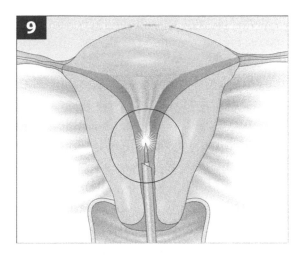

taposed fundal myometrium, as the coagulating power of the laser will also seal small arterial vessels in the fundal uterine wall.

There are some advantages of the hysteroscopic division with fiber optic lasers. Bleeding is avoided because of the coagulating power of the laser. This energy source cuts well and is easy to manipulate, perhaps more so than the resectoscope. Since there is a lack of conductivity, fluids with electrolytes can be used. However, there are some disadvantages. The laser is an expensive energy source. The possibility of back and lateral scattering makes lasers potentially damaging to the normal endometrium peripheral to the septum. Finally, lasers require special maintenance and assistance, including a laser safety officer for operating the unit. Back scattering of these fiber optic lasers can damage the retina and appropriate eye protection for the surgeon and assisting personnel is required.

Chapter 9

110 | ENDOSCOPIC TREATMENT OF UTERINE ANOMALIES . . . .

Because the procedure may be long, excessive amounts of fluids may be required. If the hysteroscope lacks a continuous flow system or double channel to collect the returning fluid after cleansing the uterine cavity from bubbles and debris, excessive fluid may be intravasated. In the absence of a perfect monitoring system for the inflow and outflow, the intravasated fluid may not be adequately measured, therefore endangering the patient with pulmonary edema secondary to fluid overload, even with the use of fluids with electrolytes. Therefore, it is important to monitor the fluid infused and maintain the intrauterine pressure so as not to exceed the mean arterial pressure of about 100 mmHg. Should excessive fluid deficit occur (more than 1500 mL) the use of diuretics should be strongly considered even though the patient is receiving normal saline.

HYSTEROSCOPIC METROPLASTY UTILIZING VAPORIZING ELECTRODES

New vaporizing bipolar electrodes, Versapoint™ (Gynecare) may also be used to divide the uterine septum (Figure 10). The technique does not vary from that of electrosurgery or lasers, but has the advantage of using fluids with electrolytes such as normal saline, therefore increasing the threshold for fluid overload and avoiding possible acute intraoperative and postoperative hyponatremia.

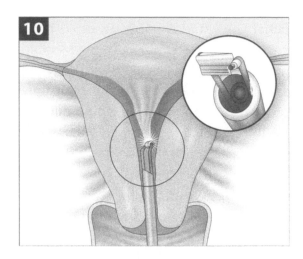

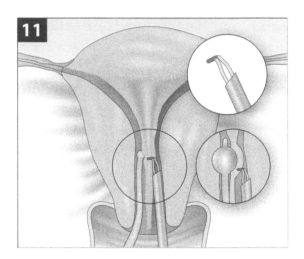

HYSTEROSCOPIC TREATMENT OF A COMPLETE UTERINE SEPTA INVOLVING THE CERVIX

The hysteroscopic treatment of this anomaly has also been established. A uterine probe or an indwelling catheter is introduced on one side of the divided cervical canal, once the opposite canal has been dilated to introduce an operative hysteroscope (Figures 11). The probe or indwelling catheter is placed just above the internal os to obtain a slight indentation of the septum at this level. Under hysteroscopic view, a small fenestration is made with semi rigid hysteroscopic scissors or other energy source, such as laser, vaporizing electrodes, or the resectoscope. The probe is inserted into the window, or the indwelling catheter is permitted to protrude slightly. When sufficient space is created to observe the opposite uterine cavity, the probe or the indwelling catheter is withdrawn. The corresponding endocervical canal is occluded with a tenaculum or the indwelling catheter is slightly deflated to occlude the cervical canal. The hysteroscopic division of the corporeal uterine septum is then performed in the usual manner (Figure 12).

Another method has been proposed to divide the complete uterine septum with a septate cervix by performing bilateral cervical dilatation of both cervices with a No. 6 Hegar dilator. Straight Mayo scissors are used to cut 2–3 cm in the cervix permitting the insertion of the operative hysteroscope or resectoscope; the division of the corporeal septum is completed in the usual fashion (Figure 13). While this method is simple, the surgeon should be prepared if cervical bleeding occurs. The cutting should be maintained in the midline to avoid cervical injury. At the completion of the hysteroscopic/resectoscopic division of the septum, the resectoscope is withdrawn and the cervix is checked for

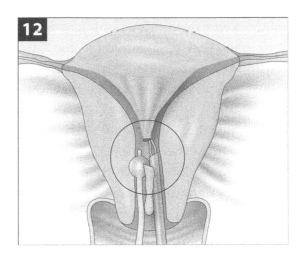

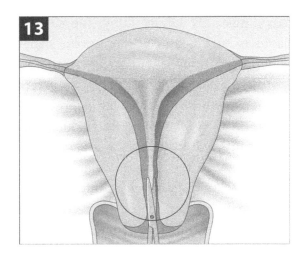

possible bleeding. Any bleeding points are coagulated.

ENDOSCOPIC TREATMENT OF THE BICORNUATE UTERUS

The bicornuate uterus may produce problems in reproduction, such as repetitive abortions, fetal malpositions, and premature labor. In the past an abdominal metroplasty by the Strassman method was used to treat this condition. This consisted of laparotomy and hysterotomy with a fundal, transverse incision from cornu to cornu. Repairs were made in layers in the anterior-posterior plane. Recently, endoscopes have been used for this endoscopic surgery. Under laparoscopic view the myometrial lining of the indenting defect of the bicornuate uterus is divided with an electrical knife through the resectoscope, sparing the serosal layer (Figure 14). This is performed about 1 cm away from the tubal openings. By laparoscopy, the serosal layer is cut utilizing a monopolar sharp electrode about 1 cm away from the cornual regions (Figure 15). The defect is then repaired in an anterior-posterior plane in one or two layers (Figure 16). Alternatively, because this repair may be difficult with the tools available today for laparoscopic suturing, a mini-laparotomy may be performed to accomplish this repair in layers. While this technique is appealing, little experience exists in its performance, not only because of the rare necessity to perform metroplasties in bicornuate uteri, but also because of the difficulty in repairing the defect endoscopically. Additionally, even if mini-laparotomy is to be performed, from a practical standpoint, it is better to initiate and complete the metroplasty through this small incision.

All endoscopic procedures at present are performed under video monitoring, not only because of the additional mag-

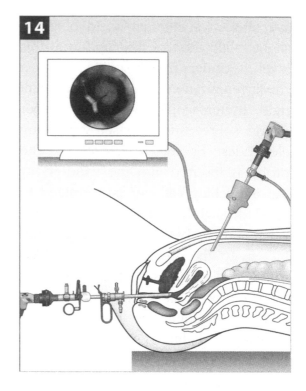

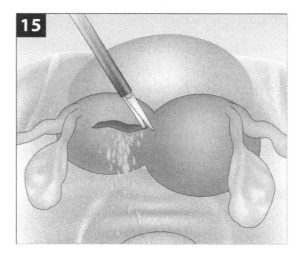

nification obtained, but also for comfort of the surgeon and the assisting personnel. Furthermore, good documentation is obtained for future review by video taping the procedures.

INTRAOPERATIVE AND POSTOPERATIVE MANAGEMENT

While it continues to be debatable, the use of prophylactic antibiotics is optional and can be used intraoperatively with cephalosporins or doxycycline. Similarly, the use of high doses of estrogen continues to be controversial, but this medication may allow a faster re-epithelialization of the denuded area left by the division of the septum. High doses of natural estrogens such as Premarin 2.5 mg twice a day orally for 30 days can be used and terminal progesterone added in the form of Provera 10 mg a day in the last ten days of this artificial cycle. It is not known whether this postoperative medical therapy benefits reproductive outcome, but some sonographic evidence exists that the endometrium thickens faster while on this regimen, therefore allowing resumption of normal endogenous hormones completing healing.

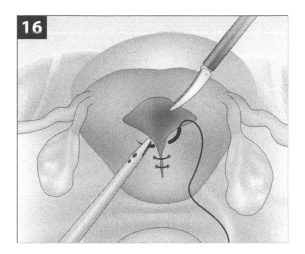

When this hormonal treatment is concluded, the uterus should be evaluated to rule out significant remnants of the septum that may require additional treatment. A hysterosalpingogram or sonography is used to assess the postoperative shape of the uterine cavity. A small, less than 1 cm remnant of the septum may not require additional treatment as clinically it has been shown that no untoward reproductive sequelae may follow.

SUGGESTED READING:

Buttram VC, Gibbons WE: Mullerian anomalies: A proposed classification (an analysis of 144 cases). Fertil Steril 1979;32:40-46

Valle RF: Hysteroscopic treatment of partial and complete uterine septum. Int J Fertil and Menop Studies 1996;41:310-315

Homer HA, Li E-C, Cooke ID: The septate uterus: a review of management and reproductive outcome. Fertil Steril 2000;73:1-14

CANNULATION OF THE FALLOPIAN TUBE

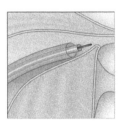

Joseph S. Sanfilippo, M.D., M.B.A.
Jonathon Solnik, M.D.

INTRODUCTION

Selective salpingography using specialized catheters under fluoroscopy has become increasingly popular for both tubal sterilization and the evaluation of tubal patency and pathophysiology. Transcervical tubal cannulation by hysteroscopic, fluoroscopic, and ultrasonographic methods are presently the most minimally invasive options for patients with infertility and proximal tubal occlusion. Approximately 20–50% of female infertility is associated with tubal obstruction, of which 20% is due to proximal disease. In the past, these patients were treated with extensive reconstructive surgery involving uterotubal implantation. Subsequent tubal patency rates ranged from 30–50% utilizing macrosurgical technique; however, the term delivery rate was unacceptably low. In 1977, microsurgical anastomosis was described. Prior to Assisted Reproductive Technologies (ART), it had been considered the gold standard for the surgical treatment of proximal tubal occlusion, yielding significantly higher, yet unreliable, term pregnancy rates. Consequently, the wide range of success with surgical interventions, compounded by the high cost of ART, mandated the need for accessible yet less invasive technologies.

With the advent of modern fiber optics, radiographic and catheter technologies, tubal cannulation has been reintroduced as a viable option for both diagnostic and therapeutic interventions.

INDICATIONS

ANATOMY

A comprehensive appreciation of the anatomy and physiology of the oviduct is essential when devising treatment options for patients with infertility and tubal disease. The oviduct typically measures 7–14 cm in length and consists of mucosal, muscular, and serosal layers (Figure 1). The muscularis is arranged in two layers of smooth muscle. The inner layer is circular and the outer is longitudinal. The intramural portion of the oviduct typically measures 1.5–2.5 cm in length with a mean diameter of 100 μm. The pathway is frequently tortuous, and successful cannulation requires a soft catheter or guide wire (Figure 2). No specific histological sphincter has been identified. This area of the tube, which is the portal for gametes to the endometrial cavity, is quite vascular and is profoundly influenced by hormonal, pharmacologic and neurologic stimuli.

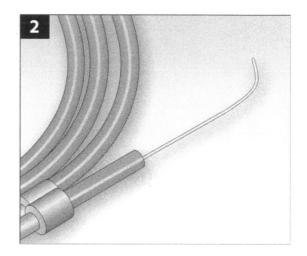

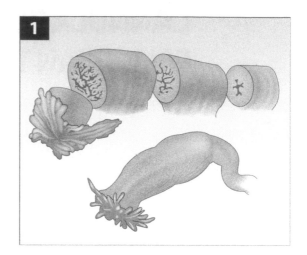

DIAGNOSTICS

Although hysterosalpingography (HSG) remains the screening method of choice for tubal occlusion, false positive rates of 20–30% may be encountered. Possible etiologies to explain these high rates include temporary events such as spasm at the uterotubal junction and mechanical obstruction from amorphous deposition. Antispasmodic agents have been of little clinical significance. Sulak performed histologic sampling of proximal tubal segments in patients undergoing microsurgical treatment for proximal occlusion demonstrated by HSG and chromopertubation. No occlusion was demonstrated in 61% of these patients. Amorphous material was found in one-third of those who did not have a true occlusion. This suggests that a significant number of patients who would otherwise undergo a major intervention for suspected occlusive disease may be appropriately diagnosed and effectively treated with a less morbid procedure. Re-establishing tubal patency may not result in subsequent pregnancy because of surgically induced intraluminal adhesion formation or inherent tubal pathology such as fibrosis or salpingitis isthmica nodosa (SIN). The desired outcome of a diagnostic study, therefore, should be to accurately diagnose true occlusion. Selective salpingography with tubal cannulation has been proposed as an alternative method to distinguishing a false obstruction from a true occlusion, boosting canalization rates of up to 85% of obstructed tubes.

HYSTEROSCOPIC CANNULATION

Patients treated with hysteroscopic cannulation show total pregnancy rates, ongoing, and ectopic rates between 29–71.4%, 29–57%, and 3.6–5.9%, respectively. These rates were not significantly different from those treated with traditional microsurgery or when compared to different techniques.

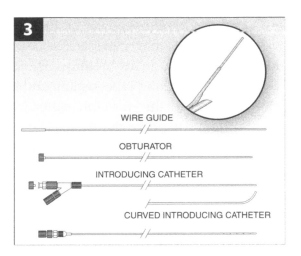

WIRE GUIDE

OBTURATOR

INTRODUCING CATHETER

CURVED INTRODUCING CATHETER

PROCEDURES:

• The patient is initially placed in the dorsal supine position until successful anesthesia has been obtained.

• The legs are then positioned in stirrups as with any hysteroscopic procedure.

• Moderate sedation with a paracervical block is well tolerated.

• The cervix is grasped with a single-toothed tenaculum and dilated sequentially to a 21 French Pratt dilator.

• Any rigid hysteroscope (12°) with an operating port may be used for the procedure.

• Catheter selection depends on preference and comfort of the operator; however, traditional catheters are based on a co-axial system (tube within a tube) (Figure 3).

• The tubal cannulation procedure is initiated with laparoscopy and conducted hysteroscopically under direct laparoscopic control (Figure 4).

• Diagnostic hysteroscopy is performed using liquid distention media (NaCl or Ringer's solution). The hysteroscope is advanced toward the tubal ostium and it can be fixed in this position either by the assistant's hand or the hysteroscope holder that is attached to the operating table, enabling the surgeon to perform the catheterization with both hands.

• The uterine catheter straightened by the inserted mandrel is introduced through the working channel of the hysteroscope.

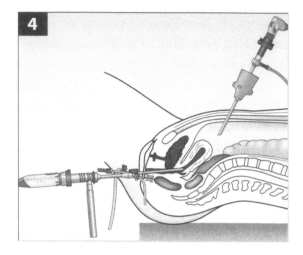

• The mandrel is then pulled out of the uterine catheter allowing the catheter to retain its curved shape pointing toward the tubal ostium (Figure 5). Under hysteroscopic guidance the uterine catheter is positioned in front of the tubal ostium. The catheter should not be advanced into the tubal ostium since it may cause injury. The role of the uterine catheter is to prevent any bending or twisting of the tubal catheter inside the uterine cavity.

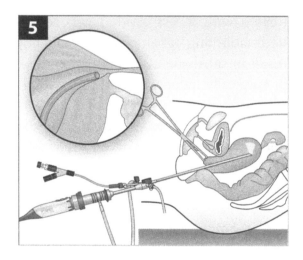

• The next step is to introduce the fallopian tube catheter through the uterine catheter and into the tubal ostium. Initially the guide wire is placed and advanced into the tubal catheter until the distal ends of the guide wire and the tubal catheter are flush in a tip to tip position. The flexibility of the guide wire is determined by the length protruding from the inner catheter. The further it extends, the more flexible it becomes. At this position, the valve is locked at the proximal end of the catheter so that the tubal catheter with inserted guide wire can be advanced into the tube under hysteroscopic and laparoscopic control (Figure 6). As soon as the catheter enters the intramural section, the hysteroscopic distention medium is turned off to prevent the liquid overdistention of the fallopian tube. The falloposcopy pump should be used to continuously irrigate the tube with Ringer's solution during the catheterization (Figure 7). When the fallopian tube catheter is advanced into the isthmic portion of the tube, the diagnostic medium of choice may be administered to evaluate for tubal patency (Figure 8). Plain film imaging requires a contrast medium; however, adequate intracavitary pressures must be maintained to avoid reflux of contrast into the vagina. Leakage of material could contribute to a higher false-positive rate. Radiation exposure may be avoided by using indigo carmine or methylene blue to assess for tubal patency. Concomitant laparoscopy must then be performed. However, the dual procedure may prove beneficial for the treatment of infertility if tubo-ovarian adhesions are noted and lysed. This requires the use of general anesthesia. Honore published data on their own series of hysteroscopic cannulation and categorized patients based on the presence or absence of pelvic adhesions. They reported no significant difference in ability to cannulate the oviduct or achieve subsequent pregnancy.

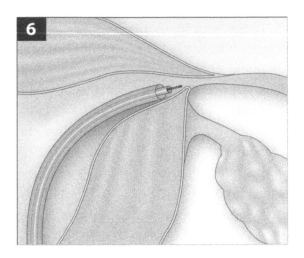

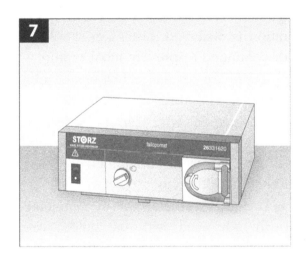

If resistance is met while advancing the guide wire, despite attempts to adjust the length of exposed guide wire, place the tapered end of the inner 3 Fr catheter into the isthmic portion of the tube. If continued resistance is encountered, then abort the procedure and attempt cannulation of the opposite tube. Remember that the majority of tubes may be cannulated; however, approximately 15% will be truly occluded by a chronic process such as SIN. Although high success rates have been reported, reocclusion may occur at a rate of 20–30%.

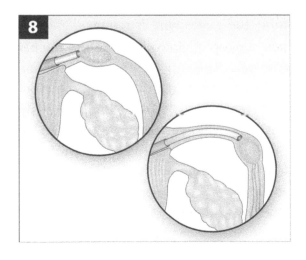

Laparoscopic monitoring of the fallopian tube catheter tip advancement is essential to prevent the overdistension and perforation or rupture of the occluded tube (Figure 9). The falloposcopy pump is connected with the catheter tubing set. The tubing must be completely filled with Ringer's solution at all times, and care must be taken to prevent air or other gases from entering the system. If the tube is occluded, extra care and caution should be taken to prevent tubal rupture by excessive pressure. If tubal wall dissection or partial perforation is observed, distention should be discontinued to prevent tubal rupture.

There are several techniques of tubal cannulation that may be performed:

• The guide wire can be advanced through the entire tube, and the tubal catheter is advanced through the tubal lumen over the guide wire.

• The tubal catheter can be simultaneously advanced with the guide wire, with the tips of the wire and the catheter being flush with each other.

• After the catheter is positioned in the tube, the guide wire is removed and the falloposcope is introduced into the tubal catheter. The tip of the falloposcope should be flush with the tip of the tubal catheter. They are simultaneously advanced allowing the visualization of the tube as the catheter is advanced toward the fimbria (Figure 10).

• Other technologies utilize the linear everting catheter. A soft, flexible membrane unrolls within the lumen of the

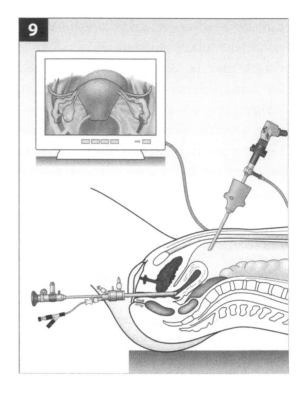

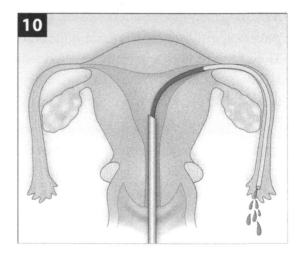

fallopian tube, obviating the need for a guide wire. This membrane consists of a catheter within a catheter fused at the distal tip, which gently dilates the tube in a circumferential manner and is useful for accommodating falloposcopes. The outer and inner catheters measure 1.2 mm and 0.7 mm in diameter, respectively (Figure 11).

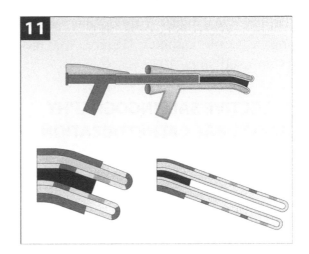

- A 5 mm flexible hysteroscope with a 2 mm operating channel may be used in a similar fashion with the use of a 1 mm catheter and guide wire. The catheter is advanced 1–2 cm into the isthmus under laparoscopic guidance, at which point, indigo carmine is injected (Figure 12). This system is especially useful when the cornua are tortuous and unreachable with a rigid scope. Flexible hysteroscopes have a flushing system to allow for a clear view of the endometrial cavity. As with a rigid hysteroscope, any distension medium may be used, including carbon dioxide. Since these procedures do not require electrocautery, we advocate the use of isotonic crystalloid solutions to avoid risk of fluid overload and hyponatremia.

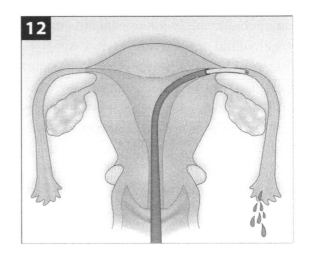

- Prophylactic antibiotics may be used because vaginal flora may be introduced into the endometrial cavity. First generation cephalosporins have been advocated; however, there is no evidence to support routine use.

- Cornual perforation is the most common complication with an incidence of 3–11%. It generally requires no intervention and the tube heals spontaneously without sequelae. Pregnancies have been reported after perforation in patients with a single functioning tube. To minimize the risk of this complication, avoid vigorous manipulation of the guide wire when attempting cannulation. If the patient has a history of pelvic inflammatory disease, consider using prophylactic antibiotics.

FLUOROSCOPIC MANAGEMENT

The technique resembles a balloon angioplasty and may be successful in creating tubal patency.

Many studies indicated that a fluoroscopic approach may be effective in correcting proximal tubal occlusion.

Transcervical balloon tuboplasty, utilizing a Cook catheter (Figure 13) has been used since 1986.

SELECTIVE SALPINGOGRAPHY AND TUBAL CATHETERIZATION

A number of catheter systems are available for selective salpingography and tubal catheterization. The Cook Ob/Gyn (Spencer, Indiana) system utilizes a balloon cervical cannula which occludes the internal cervical os with a smaller silicone balloon to maintain contrast within the uterine cavity. A 5.5 Fr Beacon™ Tip torque control outer catheter may be passed through the central channel of the cervical access catheter. The tip of this catheter is highly visible under fluoroscopy and is advanced until the tubal ostium is reached. Rapid, short injections of contrast are then administered to confirm placement and may, in turn, demonstrate tubal patency.

Utilizing a transcervical approach under fluoroscopic guidance, catheterization could be accomplished with the following technique:

A Cervical Access Catheter is placed into the uterine cavity and the balloon tip is inflated to create the tight seal around the cervical ostium (Figure 13). A series of coaxial catheters with guide wires are introduced through the cervical access catheter into the uterine cornua.

Conventional hysterosalpingography is performed using 10 mL of a diluted

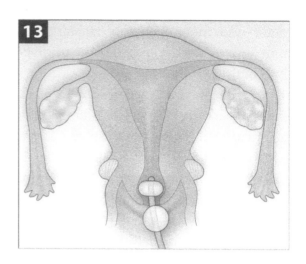

water-soluble contrast agent. A coaxial catheter system, which includes a 6 Fr Uterine Ostial Access Catheter is advanced into the uterine cavity and positioned toward the tubal ostium (Figure 14). This catheter has an atraumatic, radiopaque tip that permits visualization so the physician is aware of the location of the catheter tip. A directional indicator at the distal end of the catheter enables the physician to navigate the catheter toward the left or right fallopian tube.

If difficulty is encountered with the inner catheter, a Roadrunner® hydrophilic guidewire (.035 inch) may be substituted to facilitate penetration with minimal trauma. If proximal tubal obstruction persists, this device is advanced into the fallopian tube and is often successful in recanalizing the obstructed fallopian tube.

Once the guidewire passes the obstruction, the guidewire is removed. Alternatively, a 3 Fr translucent inner catheter is advanced through the 5.5 Fr outer catheter to and beyond the tubal ostium (Figure 15). Contrast medium is injected during this process and may demonstrate or result in tubal patency. Following cannulation, hysterosalpingography is performed in the usual manner. Patients undergoing selective catheterization should receive prophylactic antibiotics preceding the procedure.

Another version of the fluoroscopic catheter system may be used with Albumex by placing a 9 Fr balloon cervical access catheter. A 6 Fr uterine ostial access catheter is then advanced to the tubal ostium and contrast medium is injected to attest patency. The entire procedure is accomplished under ultrasound guidance.

Overall, 85% of proximal tubal obstruction can be overcome with a selective salpingography-tubal catheterization technique. Perforation is uncommon occurring in 3%–11% of patients undergoing tubal cannulation.

In patients who have undergone reversal of previous tubal sterilization with a subsequent finding of tubal occlusion, selective salpingography and tubal cannulation has been successful in correcting the obstruction at the site of anastomosis. Specifically, in a series of 38 reanastomosed fallopian tubes, patency was accomplished in 68% with use of selective salpingography-cannulation of the obstructed fallopian tube.

Studies have attested to the overall low radiation exposure with both hys-

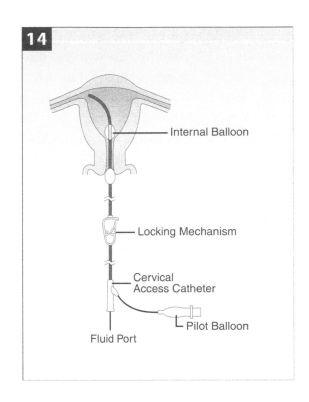

14
- Internal Balloon
- Locking Mechanism
- Cervical Access Catheter
- Pilot Balloon
- Fluid Port

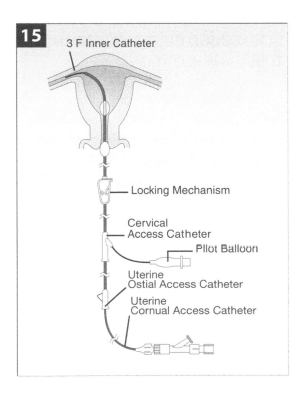

15
3 F Inner Catheter
- Locking Mechanism
- Cervical Access Catheter
- Pilot Balloon
- Uterine Ostial Access Catheter
- Uterine Cornual Access Catheter

terosalpingography as well as tubal cannulation. Specifically, assessment during selective salpingography has been associated with a dose area product-radiation exposure of 77.5 cGy CM2. In essence, this is equated with a minimal increase in long term risks of cancer of the reproductive organs.

ALTERNATIVES FOR PROXIMAL TUBAL OBSTRUCTION

DATA FROM RADIOGRAPHIC SERIES

Confino and colleagues reported a pregnancy rate of 36% (23 of 64 patients) with a transcervical balloon tuboplasty. Of these pregnancies, 1.6% were ectopic. Pregnancy rates as high as 30–50% following tubal catheterization have been reported.

ULTRASOUND GUIDED FALLOPIAN TUBE CANNULIZATION

Proximal obstruction accounts for approximately 15% of tubal disease; tubal patency rates of 90% with use of radiological procedures to "open" the occlusion and pregnancy rates of 30-40% demonstrate that alternative methods bear consideration. One such alternative is ultrasound with an ultrasound contrast agent, Albumex (Mallinkrovt Medicals, St. Louis, MO). Proximal tubal occlusion addressed under ultrasound guidance with use of an ultrasound contrast agent consisting of air-filled microspheres encased by albumin appears to

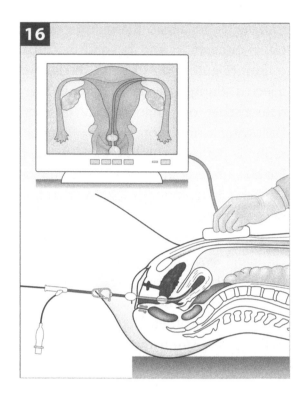

be echogenic on ultrasound. This allows for placement of a 9 Fr cervical access catheter with a 3 mL balloon. This was followed by the introduction of a 6 F uterine ostial access catheter allowing for selective catheterization of the fallopian tube then followed by injection of contrast medium attesting to patency – all of which were accomplished by ultrasound techniques (Figure 16).

Other ultrasound-guided techniques have utilized saline solution for assessment of proximal tubal occlusion. Ultrasound affords less radiation exposure but is often technically more challenging though less costly. It has been reported that patency in at least one side was accomplished in 84.2% of patients. Six of fourteen tubes (43%) were noted to reocclude. Alternative approaches to proximal tubal occlusions include a microsurgical approach with resection of the occluded proximal segment of fallopian tube. In the majority of cases, a segment of intramural, i.e., within the uterine segment of the tube, can be identified for reanastomosis. Other alternatives include assisted reproductive technology with the ability to bypass the fallopian tubes and transfer an embryo directly into the uterine cavity.

TUBAL PERFUSION PRESSURES

One report has attested to patients with endometriosis having elevated tubal perfusion pressures compared with those without disease. The higher tubal perfusion pressure was equated with tubal occlusion that was noted during hysterosalpingography-selective salpingography. Work reported by Karande et al. measured tubal perfusion pressures during selective salpingography. Elevated tubal perfusion pressures >350 mmHg were noted in 22 patients with endometriosis. Normal tubal perfusion pressures, <350 mmHg, were noted with a normal pelvis. Other pathologic problems equated with elevated tubal perfusion include salpingitis isthmica nodosa as well as tubal adhesions. The authors hypothesized that elevated tubal perfusion pressure precluded the occurrence of pregnancy.

Chapter 10

126 | **CANNULATION OF THE FALLOPIAN TUBE** ···

SUGGESTED READING:

Flood JT, Grow DR. Transcervical tubal cannulation: a review.
Obstet Gynecol Surv 1993;48:768-76

Honore GM, Holden AEC, Schenken RS. Pathophysiology and management
of proximal tubal blockage. Fertil Steril 1999;71(5):785-95

Risquez F, Confino E. Transcervical tubal cannulation, past, present, and future.
Fertil Steril 1993;60(2):211-26

Valle RF. Tubal Cannulation. Obstet Gynecol Clin No Amer 1995;22(3):519-40

Rouanet JP, Chalalut J. An application of selective catheterization: salpingography.
Nouv Presse Med 1977;Sept 24;6(31):2785

Platia N, Krudy A. Transvaginal fluoroscopically recanalization of a proximally
occluded oviduct. Fertil Steril 1985;44:704-6

Confino E, Friberg J, Gleicher N. Transcervical balloon tuboplasty. Fertil Steril
1986;46:963-6

Thurmond A, Brandt K, Gorrill N. Tubal obstruction after ligation
reversal surgery: Results of catheter recanalization. Radiology 1999;210-747-753

Shiekh H, Yussman M. Radiation exposure of ovaries during hysterosalpingography,
Am J Obstet Gynecol 1976;124:307-310

Papaioannou S, Afnan M, Coomarasamy A, Ola B, Hammadieh N, Temperton D,
McHugo J, Sharif K. Long-term safety of fluoroscopically guided selective salpingography
and tubal catheterization. Hum Repro Feb 2002;7:370-372

Confino E, Han T, Gleicher N. Sonographic transcervical balloon tuboplasty.
Hum Repro 1992;7:1271-3

Hepp H, Torell N, Strowitzki T. Proximal tubal obstruction-Is there a best way?
Hum Repro 1996;11:1823-1834

Confino E, Tur-Kaspa I, DeChernui A, Corfam R, Coulam C, Robinson E. Transcervical
balloon tuboplasty. A multicenter study. JAMA 1990;246:2079-82

Lisse K, Sybow P. Fallopian tube catheterization and recanalization under ultrasonic
observation: a simplified technique to evaluate tubal patency and open proximally
obstructed tubes. Fertil Steril 1991;56:198-201

Karande VC, Pratt DE, Rao R, Balin M, Gleicher N. Elevated tubal perfusion pressures
during selective salpingography are highly suggestive of tubal endometriosis. Fertil Steril
Dec 1995;64:1070-3

Karande VC, Pratt DE, Rabin DS, Gleicher N. The limited value of hysterosalpingography in assessing tubal status and fertility potential. Fertil Steril 1995;63:1167-71

HYSTEROSCOPIC TUBAL STERILIZATION

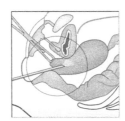

Jay M. Cooper, M.D.

INTRODUCTION

A transcervical approach to tubal sterilization offers a non-incisional alternative to laparoscopic surgery that eliminates the need for general anesthesia and that can be readily adapted to an outpatient or office setting. Benefits of this less invasive approach include reduced postprocedure pain, allowing a patient to resume normal activities more quickly.

A transcervical approach could be especially valuable when laparoscopic surgery is contraindicated, e.g., in women who are obese, have severe cardiopulmonary dysfunction or diaphragmatic hernia, or have previously undergone abdominal/pelvic surgery.

A system that employs a hysteroscopic approach for non-incisional tubal sterilization has recently been developed and shown in clinical trials to be safe and effective. The Essure® (Conceptus, Inc.) permanent birth control system consists of a micro-insert, a disposable delivery system, and a disposable split introducer (Figure 1). A standard hysteroscope employing continuous flow technology with a 5 Fr working channel and a 12°–30° angled lens is used with the system. The micro-insert consists of a stainless steel inner coil, a nitinol outer coil and polyethylene terephthalate (PET) fibers that are wound in and around the inner coil. The micro-insert is 4 cm in length and 0.8 mm in diameter in its wound down configuration (Figure 2A). When released, the outer coil expands to 1.5 to 2.0 mm (Figure 2B). One micro-insert is placed in the proximal section of each fallopian tube lumen. When the micro-insert expands upon release, it acutely anchors itself in the endosalpingeal mucosa, spanning the uterotubal junction. Permanent birth control is subsequently achieved when tissue in-growth into the micro-insert permanently anchors the micro-insert and occludes the fallopian tube. A hysterosalpingogram (HSG) is performed 3 months after micro-insert placement to evaluate tubal occlusion. Once tubal occlusion is confirmed, patients are able to rely on the micro-inserts for permanent contraception.

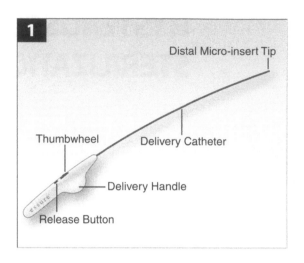

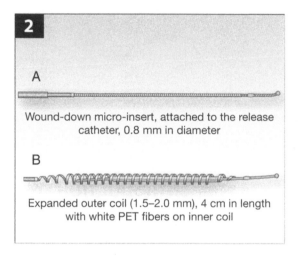

Wound-down micro-insert, attached to the release catheter, 0.8 mm in diameter

Expanded outer coil (1.5–2.0 mm), 4 cm in length with white PET fibers on inner coil

PATIENT SELECTION, PREPARATION AND POSITIONING

This system is intended for interval tubal sterilization in women who are at least 6 weeks past delivery or for termination of a pregnancy. Micro-insert placement should be performed during the early proliferative phase of the menstrual cycle in order to both decrease the potential for micro-insert placement in a patient with an undiagnosed (luteal phase) pregnancy and enhance visualization of the fallopian tube ostia. Micro-insert placement should not be performed during menstruation.

This procedure should be considered irreversible and therefore candidates must be certain about their desire to end fertility. Patients must also have two patent fallopian tubes and no active or recent upper or lower pelvic infections. Contraindications to micro-insert placement include pregnancy or suspected pregnancy, known reproductive tract abnormalities, and known allergy to contrast media or known hypersensitivity to nickel confirmed by skin testing.

A pregnancy test should be conducted within 24 hours prior to the micro-insert placement procedure. The patient must use an alternative form of contraception (except an intrauterine device) following the micro-insert placement procedure until the 3-month HSG has confirmed both proper micro-insert placement and complete tubal occlusion. It is important to ensure that the patient is supplied with, or already has, contraception for this time frame.

Administration of a non-steroidal anti-inflammatory drug (NSAID) is recommended one to two hours before the micro-insert placement procedure. Administration of a local anesthetic (eg., paracervical block), is advised prior to placement of the micro-inserts. IV sedation can also be added if desired. If only a paracervical block is used, an anxiolytic agent may also be offered 30 minutes prior to the procedure to reduce anxiety.

The micro-insert placement procedure can be performed in either an outpatient or office surgery setting, and should not exceed 20 minutes (10 minutes per tube). A scrub nurse (or technician) should assist the physician in the performance of the Essure® procedure.

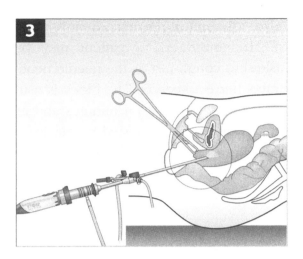

This individual may provide assistance in inserting the Essure® split introducer and the Essure® delivery system through the sealing cap of the hysteroscope working channel while the physician manipulates the hysteroscope to identify and maintain visualization of the tubal ostia.

The patient is placed in the lithotomy position and draped using standard procedures (Figure 3). An under buttocks drape with a fluid control pouch is recommended for fluid management. Ski boot style stirrups are recommended to allow for ideal patient positioning and maximum comfort. If the fallopian tubes are laterally situated, the position of the patient's legs may need to be widened to allow hysteroscopic access.

A speculum, preferably one that is bivalved and open-sided and thus easily removed, is placed in the vagina and the cervix is prepped with betadine or other suitable antibacterial solution. A paracervical block is administered. To minimize discomfort during administration of the anesthetic, a patient may be asked to cough just as the needle penetrates her ecto-cervix. The block is usually complete in 3 to 4 minutes and its effectiveness can be tested by placing a tenaculum on the anterior lip of the cervix. The patient should be unaware of this placement.

HYSTEROSCOPIC EVALUATION OF THE OSTIA

A simplified flowchart for the placement procedure is presented in Figure 4. Once the hysteroscope has been prepared and checked, the inflow port should be opened, the outflow port closed and the system (both hysteroscope and tubing) flushed of all air bubbles. The patient is informed that the hysteroscope is about to be introduced into the cervical canal and she is invited to view the procedure on the video monitor. Both physician and assistant can keep the patient informed throughout the procedure, such as explaining the anatomy seen on the video monitor.

With irrigation fluid flowing freely, the sterile hysteroscope is inserted through the cervix into the uterine cavity. The physician should be aware that the dark circle now seen on the video monitor corresponds to the not yet illuminated uterine fundus. When using a rigid hysteroscope with a 12° to 30° offset lens, the position of the light post is

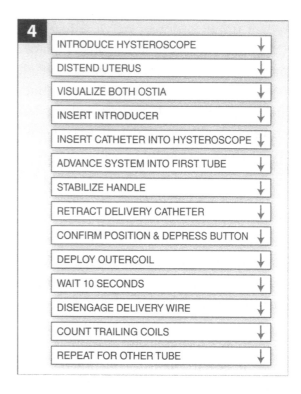

4

INTRODUCE HYSTEROSCOPE	↓
DISTEND UTERUS	↓
VISUALIZE BOTH OSTIA	↓
INSERT INTRODUCER	↓
INSERT CATHETER INTO HYSTEROSCOPE	↓
ADVANCE SYSTEM INTO FIRST TUBE	↓
STABILIZE HANDLE	↓
RETRACT DELIVERY CATHETER	↓
CONFIRM POSITION & DEPRESS BUTTON	↓
DEPLOY OUTERCOIL	↓
WAIT 10 SECONDS	↓
DISENGAGE DELIVERY WIRE	↓
COUNT TRAILING COILS	↓
REPEAT FOR OTHER TUBE	↓

opposite the field of view (See Chapter 2). This dark circle can be used as a guide to properly place the hysteroscope and advance it atraumatically through the endocervical canal into the uterus. Visual and verbal contact should be maintained with the patient during this potentially uncomfortable maneuver. The cervix should not be dilated unless necessary for hysteroscope insertion, and when necessary, the dilation should be only as much as is required to insert the hysteroscope.

The speculum is removed and the uterine cavity is distended with a 0.9% normal saline infused through the inflow channel of the hysteroscope. The saline solution should be pre-warmed to body temperature and introduced under gravity feed to minimize spasm of the fallopian tubes (Figure 5). Adequate uterine distension is essential throughout the procedure in order to allow identification of, and access to, the tubal ostia. Standard fluid monitoring should be followed throughout the procedure, and if more than 1500 cc of saline is used, the procedure should be terminated to avoid hypervolemia. Moreover, to further reduce the risk of hypervolemia, the hysteroscopic procedure time should not exceed 20 minutes.

Both tubal ostia should be assessed hysteroscopically prior to proceeding with the micro-insert placement procedure. If it appears unlikely that successful bilateral micro-insert placement can be achieved because of uterine or fallopian tube anomalies, then the procedure should be halted.

MICRO-INSERT PLACEMENT

Once the fallopian tube ostia have been identified and judged to be suitable, the Essure® system is removed from its sterile packaging and the split introducer (with the opening face-up) is inserted through the sealing cap on the hysteroscope working channel. Prior insertion of the split introducer prevents damage from occurring to the micro-insert as it passes through the sealing cap of the hysteroscope working channel. It is important to remember to keep the hysteroscope operating channel stopcock in the open position in order to prevent damage either to the micro-insert and/or introducer.

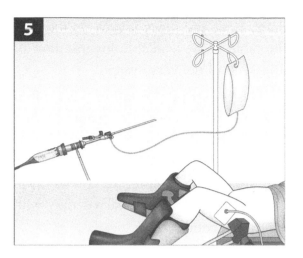

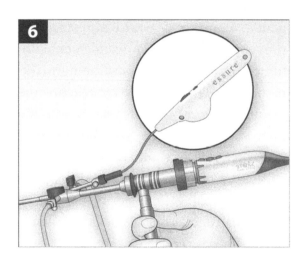

Once the stylet is removed from the split introducer, the delivery catheter is inserted through the introducer (Figure 6) and advanced through the operating channel of the hysteroscope into the uterus. The physician should gently grasp the delivery system with the thumb and forefinger so as to ease its advancement down the hysteroscope working channel. The introducer is then removed from the sealing cap, and the assistant should reload the stylet into the introducer and place it back on the sterile table to be available for insertion of the second delivery system.

Hysteroscope rotation is often required to access the ostium. When doing so, the camera head should remain still and positioned at 12 o'clock. An angled lens (either 12° or 30°) will aid in aligning the hysteroscope with the tubal ostium.

The delivery catheter is advanced into the proximal fallopian tube with gentle, constant forward movement to prevent tubal spasm. Advancement continues until the black positioning marker on the delivery catheter reaches the ostium (Figure 7). At this point, the micro-insert, hidden by the delivery catheter and constrained by the release catheter, is now spanning the intramural and proximal isthmic segments of the fallopian tube. This is the ideal placement for the micro-insert as it now spans the uterotubal junction. Advancement of the delivery system into the ostium beyond the positioning marker can lead to unsatisfactory micro-insert placement and/or tubal/uterine perforation and should be avoided.

Micro-insert placement is also acceptable when the black positioning marker cannot be advanced all the way to the tubal ostium but is at a maximum of one positioning marker length away from the tubal ostium (proximal to the ostium) (Figure 8).

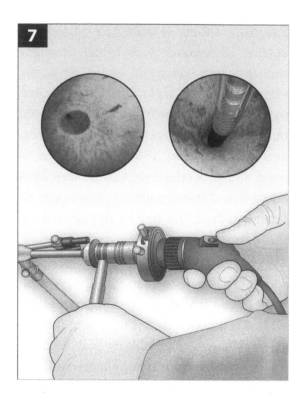

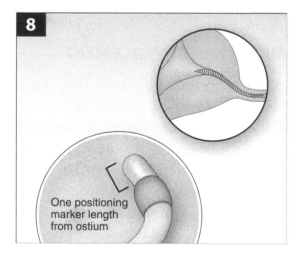

One positioning marker length from ostium

Advancing the hysteroscope as close as possible to the tubal ostium will provide additional column strength or support to the delivery catheter as it traverses the proximal tube.

The micro-insert should never be advanced if excessive resistance is encountered. Resistance to advancement manifests as: 1) the black positioning marker not advancing forward toward the tubal ostium, and/or 2) the delivery catheter bending or flexing excessively. When such resistance is observed or felt, no further attempts should be made to place the micro-insert. Such excessive resistance increases the risk of utero-tubal perforation or inadvertent placement of the micro-insert in the uterine musculature rather than within the tubal lumen. A follow-up HSG should be undertaken to determine tubal patency.

Once the delivery catheter is properly positioned, the micro-insert can be deployed, the first step of which is withdrawal of the delivery catheter. To prevent inadvertent forward movement of the micro-insert during retraction of the delivery catheter, it is important to first stabilize the handle of the Essure® micro-insert delivery system against the hysteroscope or camera while being careful not to grasp or bend the delivery catheter.

To withdraw the delivery catheter, the thumbwheel on the Essure® handle is rotated back toward the operator at a rate of 1 click per second until the wheel stops (Figure 9). The black positioning marker will be seen to move away from the tubal ostium and disappears out of view into the hysteroscope operating channel. Once thumbwheel

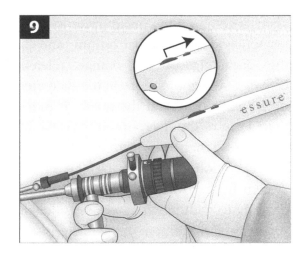

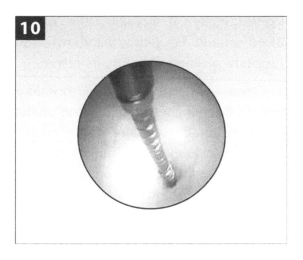

rotation begins, no attempt should be made to reposition the micro-insert until the delivery catheter is fully retracted.

The wound-down micro-insert attached to the orange release catheter can now be visualized (Figure 10). Approximately 1 cm of the wound-down coils of the micro-insert should appear trailing into the uterus. To confirm proper positioning of the micro-insert, the operator should identify two landmarks in the same field of view: 1) a small notch on the micro-insert located just outside of the tubal ostium, and 2) the distal tip of the orange release catheter. A slight increase in the diameter of the coils occurs at the notch. If more than 1 cm of the micro-insert is visible in the uterus, then the micro-insert should be repositioned by moving the entire system further into the tube before proceeding to withdraw the release catheter. A too distal placement of the micro-insert can result if the orange release catheter has been advanced into the tubal ostium. Consequently, if possible, the micro-insert should be gently withdrawn and properly positioned before its release.

Once – and only if – proper positioning has been achieved, the button on the Essure® handle is depressed to enable the thumbwheel to be further rotated. Then, while the handle continues to be stabilized against the hysteroscope, the thumbwheel is rotated back toward the operator until it cannot be rotated any further (Figure 11). This step results in the withdrawal of the orange release catheter and allows the outer coils of the micro-insert to expand. If coil expansion is not observed, the delivery wire should be gently moved away from the uterine wall so as to release pressure on the outer coil. It takes approximately 10 seconds for the outer coils of the micro-insert to expand fully, and it is important to wait until the coils are fully expanded before moving on to the last step of the procedure – disengaging and removing the delivery wire.

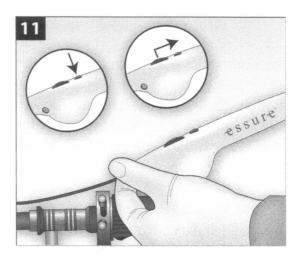

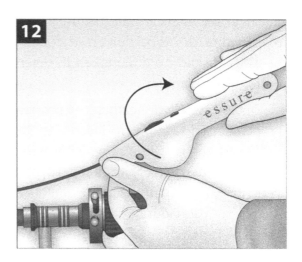

The delivery wire is disengaged from the micro-insert by rotating the entire handle counterclockwise until the delivery wire has visibly disengaged from the micro-insert (the delivery wire begins to come out from within the inner coil lumen), or until 10 full rotations of the handle have been completed, whichever comes first. While continuing to rotate the handle, the operator should gently pull the handle backward to release the delivery wire from the micro-insert (Figure 12). The delivery wire is then removed through the operating channel of the hysteroscope.

The position of the expanded micro-insert should be assessed and documented in the patient chart, along with any other issues such as poor visualization of the ostia or excessive force necessary during the placement procedure. Ideally 3 to 8 expanded outer coils of the micro-insert should be trailing into the uterus (Figure 13). If the deployed micro-insert is not properly placed, removal should not be attempted hysteroscopically as fallopian tube perforation or other patient injury could result. The only exceptions are when 18 or more coils of the micro-insert are trailing into the uterine cavity or the micro-insert has been inadvertently deployed into the uterine cavity. Because of immediate anchoring, however, removal of a micro-insert with 18 trailing coils may not be possible even immediately after placement. In such a case, surgery may be necessary to remove a malpositioned micro-insert.

The placement procedure is then repeated in the contralateral fallopian tube.

POST-PLACEMENT FOLLOW-UP

It is mandatory that patients undergo a HSG three months after the placement procedure to evaluate both micro-insert location and fallopian tube occlusion. Only if micro-insert location is satisfac-

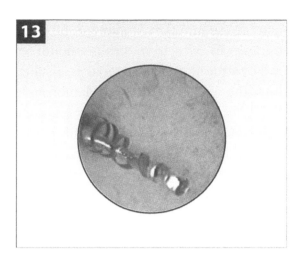

tory and there is evidence of bilateral occlusion of the fallopian tubes, should the patient be instructed to discontinue use of alternative contraception and rely on the micro-inserts for pregnancy prevention.

In order to verify that the micro-insert spans the utero-tubal junction, the uterine cavity silhouette must be clearly seen with good cornual filling and the fluoroscopy beam should provide as close to A/P projection of the uterus as possible. Dilation of the cervix should be avoided because a good cervical seal needs to be maintained throughout the procedure. It should be recognized that a correctly placed micro-insert may appear to be more distal on HSG than that which was seen at the time of hysteroscopy.

A minimum of six still radiographs should be taken to assess micro-insert location and tubal occlusion. These include: 1) a "scout film" in which the lie and curvature of the micro-inserts can be seen; 2) a minimum fill radiograph in which a small amount of radiopaque contrast material is instilled into the uterine cavity to demonstrate evidence of adequate seal of the uterine cervix (Figure 14); 3) partial fill of the uterine cavity with contrast material; 4) total fill of the uterine cavity with contrast material, the amount being determined by patient tolerance or maximal distension of the cornua, whichever comes first. The contrast material is now likely to meet or obscure the proximal (uterine) portions of the micro-inserts (Figure 15). In order to obtain a satisfactory image, additional intracavitary contrast, with a resultant increase in intrauterine pressure, is often needed. The situation should be carefully monitored to avoid undue patient discomfort and the possibility of resultant vasovagal reaction such as profound bradycardia, lightheadedness, sweating and fainting. Radiographs 5 and 6 are obtained at maximum uterine filling. They are magnified views of left and right cornua and should highlight the position of the micro-insert with respect to the cornua.

The micro-inserts have a number of radiographic markers (Figure 16), and in evaluating micro-insert position it is important to note the "markers" for the proximal end of the micro-insert (the end of the inner coil and the platinum band of the outer coil). Micro-insert position is evaluated according to its relationship to the distended uterine cornua. Measurements of these relative

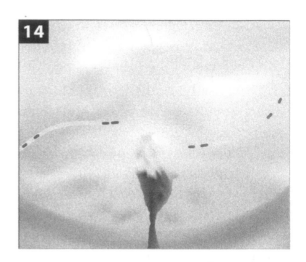

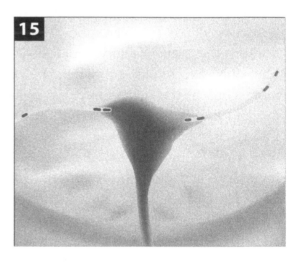

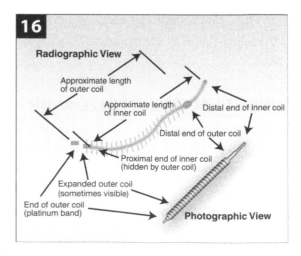

distances can be taken with a caliper. Ideal micro-insert location occurs when the inner coil of the micro-insert crosses the utero-tubal junction (Figure 8). The inner coil is the critical component for evaluation because the PET fibers that elicit fibrosis and occlusion are located on the inner coil of the micro-insert.

Satisfactory placement occurs when the distal end of the inner coil is within the fallopian tube with less than 50% of the length of the inner coil trailing into the uterine cavity, or the proximal end of the inner coil is up to 30 mm into the tube from where contrast fills the uterine cornua (Figure 17). The micro-insert is judged to have been placed too proximally if more than 50% of the length of the inner coil is trailing into the uterine cavity. Too distal placement is evidenced if the proximal end of the inner coil of the micro-insert appears to be more than 30 mm distal into the tube from the contrast filling the uterine cornua.

The most critical aspect of evaluating tubal occlusion is determining whether the contrast material is visible in the fallopian tube beyond the micro-insert. Any degree of proximal tubal filling with contrast material, even if the tube is occluded, should also be noted. If the tube is occluded at the cornua or contrast material is seen within the tube but not past any portion of the length of the outer coil of the micro-insert, the required tubal occlusion has been achieved.

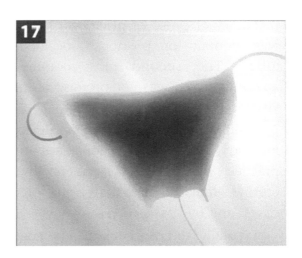

When both correct micro-insert placement and tubal occlusion have been confirmed the patient may rely on the micro-inserts for permanent contraception.

PLACEMENT SUCCESS RATE

A major obstacle to hysteroscopic tubal sterilization in the past was a low bilateral placement or occlusion rate. Placement failure can result from several circumstances: unsuspected interuterine or tubal pathology, unremitting tubal spasm, laterally positioned tubal ostia, endometrial bleeding or fragmentation, or device expulsion. In contrast to earlier attempts, the participating investigators in both Essure® clinical trials achieved a high bilateral placement rate. In the Phase II study, bilateral micro-insert placement was successful in 88% of women, while in the larger pivotal trial, it was ultimately successful in 464 (92%) of 507 women.

The chief cause of placement failure was stenotic or previously occluded tubes. The second most common anatomic cause was compromise of the visual field by the endometrium.

Training for placement of the device includes a 1-day instructional session, practice with device placement in a uterine simulator, three to five proctored cases, and five assisted cases.

Typically, the procedure can be completed in 30 minutes. In the pivotal trial, the time elapsed from hysteroscope insertion to its removal averaged 13 minutes. Following the procedure, women were quickly discharged from the recovery room (on average, after 44 minutes).

Following the procedure, vaginal bleeding is usually reported as light flow or spotting, persisting an average of 3 days. Although approximately a third of the women reported pain during the first post-procedure day, almost no one did on subsequent days.

EFFECTIVENESS AND TOLERABILITY

Long-term tolerance of the micro-insert was closely evaluated, through both interviews and diaries kept by the women. At follow-up visits, women consistently rated their tolerance for wearing the micro-insert device as "high." In the pivotal trial, 99% of women at all follow-up visits rated comfort as "good to excellent." More than 98% of women were "satisfied" or "very satisfied" at all follow-up visits.

Three months after micro-insert placement, correct device placement and bilateral tubal occlusion could be confirmed in 96% of women participating in the pivotal trial. No pregnancies have been reported in either the Phase II or pivotal trials, which taken together now total more than 10,000 women-months of follow-up. Women in the pivotal trial will be followed for 5 years to determine long-term efficacy.

SUGGESTED READING:

Cooper JM, Carignan CS, Cher D, Kerin JF. Microinsert nonincisional hysteroscopic sterilization. Obstet Gynecol 2003;102(1):59-67

Kerin JF, Carignan CS, Cher D. The safety and effectiveness of a new hysteroscopic method for permanent birth control: results of the first Essure pbc clinical study.
Aust N Z J Obstet Gynaecol 2001;41:364-370

Kerin JF, Cooper JM, Price T, Van Herendael BJ, Cayuela-Font E, Cher D, Carignan CS. Hysteroscopic sterilization using a micro-insert device: results of a multicenter phase II study. Hum Reprod 2003;18(6):1223-1230

Neuwirth RS. Update on transcervical sterilization.
Int J Gynaecol Obstet 1995;51 Suppl 1:S23-28

Valle RF, Carignan CS, Wright TC. Tissue response to the STOP microcoil transcervical permanent contraceptive device: results from a prehysterectomy study.
Fertil Steril 2001;76:974-980

HYSTEROSCOPIC MYOMECTOMY

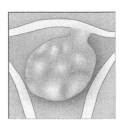

Keith B. Isaacson, M.D.
Ginger N. Cathey, M.D.

Approximately 620,000 hysterectomies were performed in the United States in 2001 with uterine leiomyomas being the most common indication. While many women have benefited from a hysterectomy that was appropriately indicated and correctly performed, it is widely believed that numerous unnecessary hysterectomies are performed each year. With greater scrutiny of hysterectomy for myomas and with various surgical and technological advancements arising, many alternatives to hysterectomy are now present. It must be recognized however that all surgical alternatives to hysterectomy allow for the possibility of new leiomyomas to form, and preexisting leiomyomas that were too small to be detected or were intentionally not removed may exhibit significant growth. For women who desire more children or want to retain their uterus and for patients who are not surgical candidates for more invasive procedures, hysterectomy alternatives should be considered. Myomectomy is one of the more common alternatives to hysterectomy. While gynecologists in this country often perform abdominal myomectomy, endoscopic myomectomy is infrequently utilized for treatment of symptomatic uterine fibroids.

Chapter 12

142 | HYSTEROSCOPIC MYOMECTOMY . . . .

Myomectomy removes only visible and accessible fibroids from the uterus. This allows the patient to retain her uterus and therefore her fertility if desired. Traditionally most myomectomies have been performed via laparotomy. Laparoscopic myomectomy and hysteroscopic myomectomy however are also options that should be considered in appropriate candidates. Laparoscopic myomectomy is best suited for removing subserosal and intramural fibroids and hysteroscopic myomectomy can be utilized to treat submucosal leiomyomas.

Today's gynecologists, however, underutilize hysteroscopy. Many gynecologists lack advanced hysteroscopic skills due to inadequate residency training and because of undue fears of the possible complications from these procedures. It is estimated that less than one-third of gynecologists in the United States perform operative hysteroscopy including hysteroscopic myomectomy. In a 1997 survey of members of the American Association of Gynecologic Laparoscopists, an organization dedicated to gynecological endoscopic surgery, only one-half of the responding members performed hysteroscopic resection of submucous fibroids. Given that this modality is minimally invasive and highly effective in treating submucous leiomyoma, it is important that this treatment option be offered to patients and that more gynecologists acquire the skills necessary to perform this procedure.

SUBMUCOUS FIBROIDS

Excessive bleeding from fibroids is most commonly due to submucosal fibroids. The volume of myoma impinging on the endometrial cavity is thought to influence the intensity of bleeding. Large, tortuous vessels often cover the endometrial surface of these tumors. It is believed that these fragile vessels are largely responsible for the menorrhagia symptoms associated with fibroids. Also, both submucosal and mucosal fibroids are believed to interfere with uterine contractility and therefore effective hemostasis may be compromised in patients with uterine leiomyomas.

While pain is most often seen with pedunculated fibroids undergoing torsion or with large degenerating fibroids, pain may also be seen in patients with a submucosal myoma protruding through the lower uterine segment causing cervical dilation. Submucosal fibroids can also interfere with implantation thereby causing infertility or they may impair blood flow to the developing embryo instigating early pregnancy loss. In addition, these myomas can block the tubal ostia impairing sperm or embryo transport through the fallopian tubes. Fortunately, evidence supports the theory that submucosal fibroids cause a decrease in fertility that is alleviated by myomectomy and with the advent of hysteroscopic resection, such fibroids can be easily removed via a relatively minor surgical procedure.

Submucosal fibroids are typically placed into one of three hysteroscopic classes based on their location in the myometrium. The Wamsteker and Block classification describes myomas as either type 0, type I or type II depending on the percentage of fibroid within the endometrial cavity; note that this classification of submucous myoma differs from that described for myomas visualized by SIS as featured in Chapter 1. A type 0 myoma is pedunculated, 100% within the cavity and therefore does not involve the myometrium (Figure 1). A type I fibroid involves the myometrium but >50% of the tumor is within the cavity (Figure 2). A type II fibroid has an intramural component that is >50% and can be transmural, located anywhere from the submucosa to the serosa. These myomas often appear as a bulge or indention in the submucosa when viewed hysteroscopically (Figure 3).

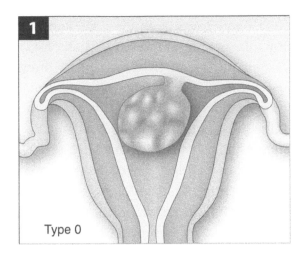

Type 0

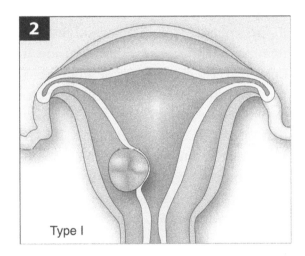

Type I

PREOPERATIVE EVALUATION

Knowing the type of submucous myoma prior to surgery is critical for planning the appropriate surgery, decision making for endometrial pretreatment, and giving the patient the appropriate expectations preoperatively. Type 0 and type I submucous fibroids are more successfully removed in one surgery whereas type II submucous myomas often require two procedures for complete removal. Hysteroscopy has

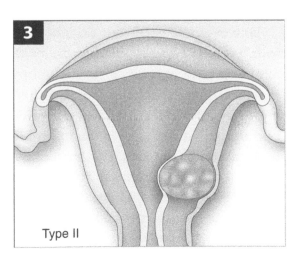

Type II

long been considered the gold standard for diagnosing intrauterine pathology. Diagnostic office hysteroscopy is often used to evaluate patients with abnormal uterine bleeding. In recent years, saline infused sonography (SIS) has become increasingly popular (see Chapter 1). Numerous studies have demonstrated that this imaging technique is far superior to standard transvaginal ultrasound and approaches hysteroscopy in correctly diagnosing intrauterine pathology. It has been suggested that SIS is as effective as hysteroscopy and well tolerated in preoperative grading of submucous myomas. The use of saline infusion to enhance visualization of the endometrium increases the diagnostic accuracy of transvaginal sonography to approach that of diagnostic hysteroscopy and is especially useful in detecting submucous fibroids. While hysteroscopy alone allows positive identification of a submucous myoma, SIS can be helpful in assessing the size of the fibroid, extent of myometrial invasion, and thickness of the overlying myometrium.

However, because we do not perform hysteroscopic myomectomies with SIS, preoperative office hysteroscopy remains the gold standard for intrauterine evaluation. This technique, when performed with a 3.1 or 3.5 mm flexible hysteroscope, requires no tenaculum, no local anesthesia and can be completed in less than one minute. The information the surgeon gathers insures there will be no surprises in the operating room since this is the same view the surgeon will see during the hysteroscopic myomectomy. The preoperative office hysteroscope provides information that can not be gathered by SIS that will affect preoperative management. Looking in the cavity allows for one to assess the vascularity of the lesion, the distention of the cavity around the myoma and the presence of additional pathology such as scar tissue that will impact preoperative planning. Since GnRH agonists have been shown to be the only medical adjuvant to reduce fluid intravasation, a look at the vascularity with the office hysteroscope can help the surgeon decide whether or not pretreatment is necessary. One can not gather this information with SIS.

Adjuvant preoperative hormonal therapy is often administered prior to hysteroscopy. It is best to perform hysteroscopic submucous myoma resection

PREOPERATIVE EVALUATION FOR HYSTEROSCOPIC MYOMECTOMY

- SALINE INFUSION SONOGRAPHY (SIS)
- HSG
- MRI
- ENDOMETRIAL BIOPSY
- HYSTEROSCOPY TO DETERMINE: LOCATION, SIZE, SHAPE, VASCULARITY

with a thin endometrium. Preoperative hormonal manipulation can assist in surgical scheduling by inducing an atrophic endometrium as opposed to waiting for the patient's follicular phase. Hysteroscopic visibility is also greatly improved with creation of an atrophic endometrium. Additionally, inducing amenorrhea and/or controlling symptoms of menorrhagia prior to surgical intervention are beneficial, especially in patients with anemia. Adjuvants that have been used for "priming" the uterus include oral contraceptives, progestins, danazol and gonadotropin releasing hormone agonist (GnRH agonist).

GnRH agonists are commonly administered prior to hysteroscopic myomectomy. Various dosing regimens exist ranging from pretreatment with Depot Luprolide Acetate 7.5 mg IM six weeks preoperatively. After the first injection, the second injection is given four weeks later and the surgery is scheduled 2–4 weeks after the second injection. Longer treatment for up to 3 months can be tried to maximize the intracavity portion of a type II myoma prior to surgery. GnRH agonists are the only drugs available that result in clinically significant uterine shrinkage and amenorrhea with maximum volume reduction occurring at 3 months of treatment. During this period of myoma volume reduction the uterus itself can shrink up to 40%, which may cause fibroids with a substantial intramural component to migrate toward the cavity. In this scenario,

myoma removal is made easier by the administration of a GnRH agonist. However, with a type II myoma that is mostly intramural, pretreatment with a GnRH agonist may result in this fibroid becoming completely intramural. Therefore, these patients should receive additional imaging prior to surgery. GnRH agonists are also advantageous in that they can reduce blood flow to the uterus and reduce fluid intravasation. Data suggests that only GnRH agonists show a statistical advantage of decreasing fluid absorption during operative hysteroscopy. One surgical disadvantage of preoperative GnRH agonists is that they may make the myoma softer and the surgical planes less distinct.

Preoperative evaluation should also consist of endometrial biopsy when indicated and the appropriate laboratory studies.

PREOPERATIVE MYOMA REDUCTION WITH GNRH-A

- INITIATE IN MID TO LATE LUTEAL PHASE
- ADMINISTER 2 DOSES
- SCHEDULE SURGERY 2–4 WEEKS AFTER 2ND INJECTION
- FOLLOW-UP WITH SIS OR OFFICE HYSTEROSCOPY BEFORE SURGERY

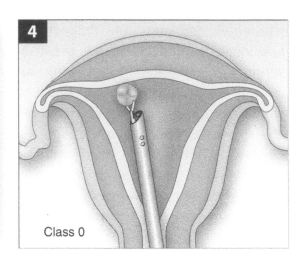

Class 0

HYSTEROSCOPIC TREATMENT OPTIONS

The goal of hysteroscopic myomectomy is removal of the entire fibroid without compromising the surrounding myometrium or endometrium. This will result in alleviation of the patient's symptoms without weakening the myometrium or creating intracavitary synechia. Removal of the entire myoma will also decrease the risk of regrowth of the lesion.

SIMPLE MYOMECTOMY

Small, pedunculated myomas can be removed simply by grasping the fibroid with polyp forceps and twisting the myoma until the stalk weakens and breaks (Figure 4). After extracting the fibroid, the base of the stalk can be examined hysteroscopically to ensure hemostasis. Larger, pedunculated, submucous leiomyomas with a thin stalk

may be removed in a similar manner, but the cervix often requires dilation to extract the fibroid from the uterine cavity. This technique should only be utilized if the fibroid is prolapsing through or to the cervix. Grabbing the fibroid blindly is not advised if the fibroid can be resected and or removed under direct visualization using either the resectoscope or the optical tenaculum.

ND:YAG LASER

During the late 1980's to the early 1990's, the Nd:YAG laser was commonly used to perform hysteroscopic myomectomies. In treating type 0 myomata, the laser is used as a cutting tool, severing the fibroid from its stalk. With other submucous leiomyomas, the laser is employed as a myolysis tool. It is used to burn several holes in the fibroid, causing devascularization and myoma shrinkage. One advantage to using this device is that it can be used

---

WHEN THE HYSTEROSCOPIC APPROACH IS NOT INDICATED

- SUBSEROSAL LESIONS ON THE ABDOMINAL SIDE OF THE UTERUS

- COMPLETELY INTRAMURAL LESIONS

- MYOMA >3 CM AND >50% INTRAMURAL EXTENSION

with an isotonic distention media. However, with the advent of other tools and accurate fluid monitoring devices, the Nd:YAG laser is rarely used for this indication today.

VERSAPOINT™ SYSTEM

The bipolar Versapoint™ system, approved by the FDA in 1996, has become more popular in recent years for treatment of submucous myomas. The Versapoint™ utilizes very high RF power (up to 200 W) to vaporize fibroids. When treating submucous fibroids with the Versapoint™, a 0°, 4 mm continuous flow hysteroscope with a 1.6 mm single fiber, spring-tip electrode is used. Alternatively, a Versapoint™ resectoscope with a 30°, 4 mm continuous flow operative hysteroscope may be used. The electrical power generator can be set to a default setting of 130 W vapor cut. The uterine cavity is distended with normal saline. With type 0 fibroids, using the spring-tip electrode may be more advantageous, resecting the fibroid at the junction with the uterine wall using a shearing technique (i.e. shaved flush with the endometrium) (Figure 5). The exposed base can then be coagulated. The free floating fibroid can be retrieved blindly with a polyp forceps or grasped under visualization with the optical tenaculum and sent for histologic assessment. The Versapoint™ resectoscope is often employed for treatment of type I and

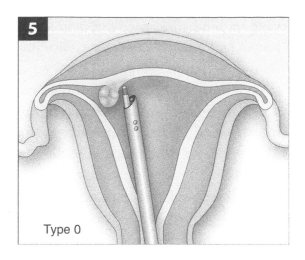

Type 0

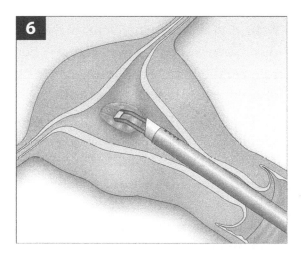

type II myomas. As the electrode is moved over the protruding fibroid instantaneous tissue vaporization and desiccation occur shaving the fibroid flush with the endometrium (Figure 6). When the uterus contracts, the remainder of the fibroid may protrude into the cavity for resection. More than one procedure may be needed for treatment of fibroids with a larger intramural component.

The Versapoint™ system has the advantage of being able to operate in isotonic fluid. The use of normal saline, however, does not preclude excessive fluid absorption. Saline is absorbed as readily as other irrigants and while there may be no electrolyte changes, pulmonary and brain edema can occur. There are also disadvantages to this system. There is no tissue sample available for pathological examination after the fibroid is vaporized. Also, the high RF of the Versapoint™ produces numerous gas bubbles. The bubbles produced by tissue vaporization can temporarily reduce visibility. Therefore, a continuous flow system is needed to help remove the bubbles. These bubbles can also enter the vascular system.

The bubbles dissipate in the blood rapidly and are usually inconsequential. However, if the rate of formation exceeds the rate of dissipation, problems could ensue. In September of 2000 Gynecare voluntarily removed Versapoint™ from the market after a small number of nonfatal gas embolisms associated with use of this system during hysteroscopic myomectomy were reported. But a panel review concluded that the risk of gas embolism with the Versapoint™ system is no greater than the risk with any other hysteroscopic electrosurgical device. Therefore it is important that the patient's end-tidal CO_2 be closely monitored throughout the procedure. If a sudden drop in end-tidal CO_2 occurs, the case should be stopped until it resolves.

MONOPOLAR LOOP ELECTRODE RESECTOSCOPE

A transcervical loop was suggested in 1957 but not until 1978 did the first report of gynecological use of a resectoscope appear. Today the resectoscope is used more than any other device in performing hysteroscopic myomectomy. The resectoscope is typically used with a 12o° telescope to allow adequate visualization of the electrode. The resectoscope is a monopolar instrument powered by high frequency alternating current. With hysteroscopic monopolar electrosurgery, low-viscosity, nonelectrolyte containing solutions should be employed. If one tried to use an isotonic electrolyte containing solution such as normal saline or lactated Ringer's, the energy at the electrode would disperse and there would be no cutting effect. Contrary to popular belief, the uterus would not be burned nor would the patient be endangered. 1.5% Glycine, 3% Sorbitol and 5% Mannitol are the 3 most commonly used uterine distention solutions with monopolar electrosurgery. It is important that the surgeon and his OR team be aware of the potential complications associated with use of these media and that fluid deficits are closely monitored during the case.

Understanding the basics of electrosurgery, one realizes that within a given range (40–100 W), little difference exists in the cutting power set on the electrosurgical generator. The principals of its use are the same. The surgeon must activate the pedal just before the loop is in contact with the tissue to be resected (Figure 7). After initiating the current, the loop must be kept moving while activated to prevent extensive thermal necrosis with a consequent risk of perforation. When using a lower wattage, more of the loop needs to be in contact with the tissue and completion of the monopolar circuit takes longer. Higher power settings allow for more rapid resection of tissue; however, only the most experienced hysteroscopic surgeon should use these settings since there is very little tactile feedback and the risk of uterine perforation is increased. The advantage of a lower power setting is that the operator has more control over the instrument. A power setting of 60 W of pure cutting current is often employed when performing hysteroscopic myomectomy. The technique for removing a submucous fibroid depends largely on its location within the endometrial cavity.

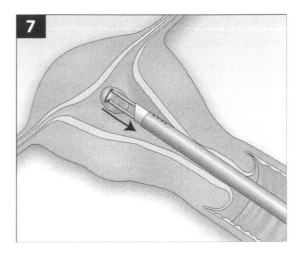

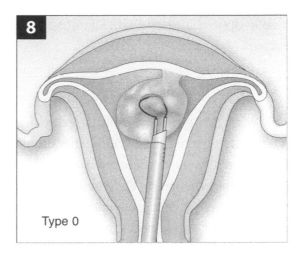

Type 0

HYSTEROSCOPIC MYOMECTOMY

- ACTIVATE BEFORE CONTACT
- ALLOW SPARK TO GENERATE ENERGY
- NEVER EXTEND AN ACTIVATED ELECTRODE
- REMEMBER CAVITY IS CURVILINEAR

TYPE 0:

As previously described, these are pedunculated intracavitary myomas. The surgeon has the option of first transecting the base of the stalk or shaving the fibroid, removing it in pieces through the cervix. For larger fibroids, it is often best to first shave the myoma (Figure 8). If the stalk is cut first, extracting a large fibroid through the cervix may prove difficult and monopolar

Chapter 12

150 | HYSTEROSCOPIC MYOMECTOMY . . . .

energy can no longer be used to cut the myoma into smaller pieces. Once the myoma is severed from the uterus the energy circuit cannot be completed. The freed fibroid can be grasped blindly with Corson forceps or under direct visualization with an Isaacson Optical Tenaculum. The cervix may have to be dilated to remove the mass. The fibroid can also be left in the cavity where it will degenerate and spontaneously be expelled. While the patient may find this last choice less desirable, it is an acceptable option and the risk of infection is low.

TYPE I:

With this type of fibroid, greater than 50% of its mass lies within the uterine cavity while the remainder is embedded in the myometrium. The resectoscope is used to shave the protruding portion of the fibroid flush with the level of the endometrium. To safely shave a submucous myoma the loop is first placed behind the fibroid to be resected. The foot pedal is then used to activate the electrosurgical energy and the loop is drawn back into the resectoscope. It is important to remember that the loop is activated before it touches the tissue. As the loop approaches the hysteroscope, maintaining visualization can be difficult. To prevent this problem, the loop, which begins its cut fully extended, is only brought halfway back to the resectoscope (Figure 9). The resecto-

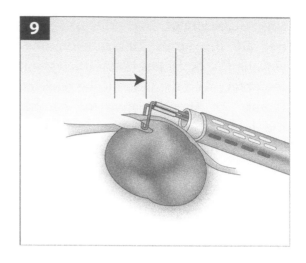

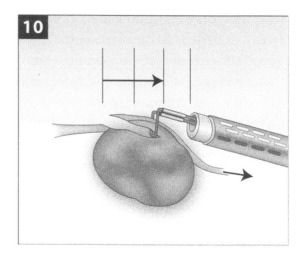

scope itself is then retracted with the loop halfway extended until the cut through the fibroid is completed (Figure 10). Additionally, as the loop is retracted into the resectoscope, the angle of the resectoscope may require adjustment to maintain contact with the fibroid.

Once the fibroid is shaved to the level of the endometrium, the myoma chips should be extracted to allow for better visualization. As the uterus contracts, more or the remainder of the fibroid may protrude into the cavity permitting its safe resection (Figure 11). When no additional fibroid extends into the cavity, the procedure is complete. This means that either complete resection of the myoma has occurred or that no additional tissue can be resected and a small amount of the fibroid remains intramural. When 70% or more of the fibroid has been removed, the remainder will usually slough off spontaneously over the next several months. If symptoms persist in these patients, the cavity can again be evaluated with SIS or preferably, the office hysteroscope.

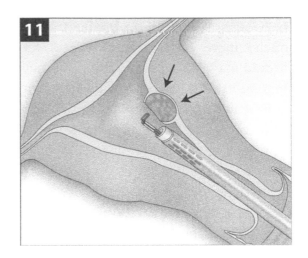

TYPE II:

Type II myomas are mostly intramural in location. They are approached in the same fashion as type I myomas. The intracavitary portion of the fibroid is first shaved to the level of the endometrium (Figure 12). Small type II myomas will often fall into the uterine cavity after this initial unroofing, making their removal easy. Larger, type II myomas however are more difficult to extract. After shaving these fibroids flush with the endometrium, the pseudo-capsular plane should be identified. The loop electrode (without energy activation) is then placed into the capsular plane and as much of the myoma as possible is retracted into the cavity (Figure 13). An optical tenaculum can also be used to twist the myoma out of the myometrial wall. The protruding portion of the fibroid is again shaved as

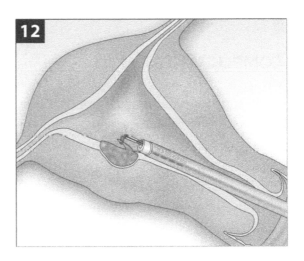

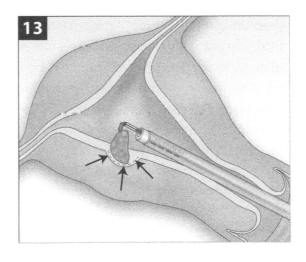

Chapter 12

152 | HYSTEROSCOPIC MYOMECTOMY . . . .

previously described. As the uterus contracts, more or the remainder of the fibroid may protrude into the cavity permitting its safe resection. This technique is repeated until all or as much as possible of the fibroid has been resected. In resecting type II submucous myomas it is advantageous to use minimal distention pressure so as to not pressure the fibroid back into the myometrium. The patient should be aware that more than one surgical attempt may be necessary for treatment of this type of myoma.

COMPLICATIONS

Hysteroscopic myomectomies, along with resection of uterine septa, are associated with a higher incidence of complications when compared to other hysteroscopic procedures. This is due to both the greater difficulty in performing these surgeries as well as the longer amount of time needed to complete the case. The primary complications encountered with hysteroscopic myoma resection are bleeding, uterine perforation, infection, and complications due to distention media. Please refer to chapter 3 to review complications related to various uterine distention media. Infection is uncommon with hysteroscopic surgery and prophylactic antibiotics are not routinely used. Infectious complications with hysteroscopy occur in 0.3–1.6% of cases and usually involve urinary tract infections, endometritis, and rarely tubo-ovarian abscesses. All patients should be questioned prior to surgery to ensure that she is not experiencing signs or symptoms of an ongoing pelvic infection.

Uterine perforation can occur during multiple steps of this procedure. Perforation may occur early on when sounding the uterus or inserting the hysteroscope. Uterine compromise can also take place later, while resecting the myoma. The surgeon must maintain constant awareness of the potential for uterine perforation and whenever a fluid deficit quickly occurs, he should consider uterine perforation. Management of uterine perforation depends on the site of injury and whether or not energy was used at the time of perforation. Perforations that occur at the fundus while using a blunt, non-energized instrument can be managed expectantly. If the site of perforation is in the lateral uterine wall or occurred with use of an energy source laparoscopy is needed to rule out broad ligament hematoma or injury to any intraperitoneal structures. With anterior perforation, cystoscopy is recommended to examine the bladder. With posterior uterine perforation, internal inspection of the colon is advised.

As with any surgical procedure, excessive bleeding is a potential complication of hysteroscopic myomectomy. Attempts to control bleeding with a rollerball are usually futile, particularly if the patient has been taken back to the

OR for postoperative hemorrhage. The intrauterine distention pressures used in hysteroscopy will usually tamponade venous bleeders, thus concealing the problem. Arterial bleeders can be seen and controlled with the rollerball, but they are less commonly a problem especially in the setting of postoperative hemorrhage (Figure 14). Postoperative bleeding is best treated with pressure and time. A 30cc Foley balloon or uterine packing with gauze soaked in a pitressin solution, left in place for 4 to 24 hours, is usually successful in tamponading the bleeders. If bleeding persists despite these efforts, uterine artery embolization should be considered prior to hysterectomy.

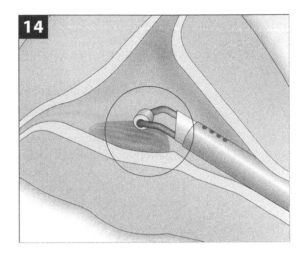

CONCLUSION

Hysteroscopic myomectomy is a highly effective and minimally invasive means of treating symptomatic submucous leiomyomas. Unfortunately, this treatment modality is underutilized by today's gynecologists. This is likely due to inadequate exposure to hysteroscopy during residency training as well as the misconception that the skills necessary to perform hysteroscopic procedures are difficult to acquire. Hopefully, with the advent of new devices, training sponsored by companies that produce these products, and with books such as this, hysteroscopy and hysteroscopic myomectomy will be more widely practiced.

SUGGESTED READING:

HCUP Nationwide Inpatient Sample (NIS), 2001, Agency for Healthcare Research and Quality (AHRQ)

Surgical Alternatives to Hysterectomy in the Management of Leiomyomas: ACOG Practice Bulletin, Number 16, May 2000

Hulka JF, Levy BS, Luciano AA, Parker WH, Phillips JM. 1997 AAGL Membership Survey: Practice Profiles, J Amer Assoc Gynecol Laparosc 1998;5:93-96

Carlson KJ, Nichols DH, Schiff I. Indications for hysterectomy. N Eng J Med 1993;328(12):856-60

Pritts E. Fibroids and infertility: A systematic review of evidence. Obstest Gynecol Survey 2001;56(8):43-491

deBlock S, Dijkman AB, Hemrika DJ. Transcervical resection of fibroids (TCRM): Results related to hysteroscopic classification. Gynaecol Endosc 1995;4:243-246

Istre O. Transcervial resection of endometrium and fibroids: the outcome of 412 operations performed over 5 years. Acta Obsterica et Gynecol Scandinavica 1996;75:567-64

Leone FP, Lanzani C, Ferrazzi E. Use of strict sonohysterographic methods for preoperative assessment of submucous myomas. Fertil Steril 2003;79(4):998-1002

Farquhar C, Ekeroma A, Furness S, Arroll B. Cochrane Menstrual Disorders and Subfertility Group. A systematic review of transvaginal ultrasonography, sonohysterography and hysteroscopy for the investigation of abnormal uterine bleeding in premenopausal women. Acta Obstetricia et Gynecologica Scandinavica. 2003;82(6):493-504

Sowter MC, Sinla AA, Lethaby A. Pre-operative endometrial thinning agents before hysteroscopic surgery for heavy menstrual bleeding: The Cochrane Database of Systemic Reviews

Donnez J, Gillerot S, Bourgonjon D, Clerckx F, Nisolle M. Neodymium: YAG laser hysteroscopy in large submucous fibroids. Fertil Steril 1990;54:999-1003

Summary Of Consensus Opinion: Scientific Panel On Gynecare Versapoint. October 15, 2000, Los Angeles, CA

Loffer F. Removal of large symptomatic intrauterine growths by the hysteroscopic resectoscope. Ob Gyn 1990;76(5)

Bradley L. Complications of hysteroscopy: prevention, treatment and legal risks. Current Opinion Ob Gyn 2002;Vol 14(4):409-415

ENDOMETRIAL ABLATION TECHNIQUES

Ginger N. Cathey, M.D.

Approximately 600,000 hysterectomies are performed each year in the United States. Abnormal or dysfunctional uterine bleeding is reported as the primary indication for surgery in 20% of these patients. With the advent of endometrial ablation, this subset of patients, about 120,000 women annually, now has a less invasive alternative to hysterectomy. Endometrial ablation is not intended to replace hysterectomy. But it does provide treatment options for both the physician and the patient. If the patient desires permanent cessation of menses, she should likely be treated with hysterectomy. But if the patient would be satisfied with lighter or normal cycles and desires to preserve her uterus or prefers a procedure with less morbidity, then endometrial ablation is an excellent alternative. Regardless of the treatment option that is chosen, women who are given a choice are more satisfied patients.

Endometrial ablation is primarily designed for the treatment of abnormal or dysfunctional uterine bleeding (AUB/DUB). This is defined as excessive uterine bleeding with no demonstrable organic cause such as fibroids, polyps, dysplasia, cancer or hematological disorders. The goal of endometrial ablation is destruction of the endometrium so as to cause decreased bleeding or even amenorrhea. The endometrium should be destroyed to the basilis level which is approximately 4–6 mm deep. Approximately 90% of patients will be successfully treated with endometrial ablation. The majority of these patients will experience decreased bleeding ranging from normal to light cycles. However, anywhere from 15–60% will develop amenorrhea depending on the endometrial technique employed.

Endometrial ablation as a treatment modality for abnormal uterine bleeding initially was not embraced by the gynecological community. First generation ablation techniques, including transcervical resection of the endometrium, rollerball ablation and laser ablation, require advanced hysteroscopic skills, distention media and the risks associated with its use, and usually general anesthesia. The technical proficiency involved in operative hysteroscopy has often intimidated the average gynecologist. Luckily, today's surgeon has available simpler means of accomplishing the same result. Second generation, global ablation techniques allow endometrial ablation to be performed easily and quickly. Most physicians become competent to perform a given technique after only 5–10 procedures. These new global ablation methods also require only basic if any hysteroscopic skills.

Advantages of performing endometrial ablation instead of hysterectomy in the appropriate candidates are numerous. Most endometrial ablations can be accomplished in less than 30 minutes as opposed to the standard 1.5 hours needed to perform a hysterectomy. Commonly, endometrial ablation can be performed with local anesthesia- paracervical block +/- IV sedation. Not only does this exempt the patient from the risks inherent in receiving general anesthesia, but it also allows physicians to treat their patient in an office setting. Endometrial ablation is an outpatient procedure whereas hysterectomy requires a hospital stay of 1–3 days. Typically, a patient that has undergone endometrial ablation can return to her regular activities the next day. Four to six weeks is the average recovery time from hysterectomy. Patients who meet the appropriate criteria for endometrial ablation should be offered this less invasive alternative for treatment of their symptoms.

INCLUSION CRITERIA

- COMPLETED CHILDBEARING
- CONTRACEPTIVES OR STERILIZATION
- NORMAL VS ABNORMAL ENDOMETRIAL CAVITY

EXCLUSION CRITERIA

- ABNORMAL PAP OR ENDOMETRIAL PATHOLOGY
- IRREGULAR CAVITY/LARGE UTERUS
- LARGE FIBROID/POLYP (>4 CM)
- PREVIOUS UTERINE SURGERY
- COMPLETE SEPTATE OR BICORNUATE UTERUS

POST ABLATION PATIENT MANAGEMENT

- CRAMPS AFTER ABLATION USUALLY 4–6 HRS (<24 HRS), BEST TREATED WITH NSAIDS
- INFECTION: RARE
- VAGINAL DISCHARGE X SEVERAL WEEKS
- CERVICAL STENOSIS & HEMATOMETRA
- ENDOMETRIAL SLOUGHING AT 3–6 MONTHS POST-OP
- STERILIZATION OR CONTRACEPTIVES

PREOPERATIVE PREPARATION

- PAP
- ENDOMETRIAL BIOPSY
- PELVIC ULTRASOUND–PREFERABLY SIS
- HYSTEROSCOPY
- GNRH AGONIST VS CURETTAGE VS NOTHING
- PREGNANCY TEST ON DAY OF PROCEDURE

ENDOMETRIAL RESECTION

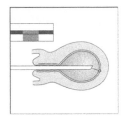

Hervé Fernandez, M.D.

INTRODUCTION

Operative hysteroscopy has modified the surgical management of benign uterine neoplasms. The first endo-uterine procedures using a resectoscope were performed for uterine malformations and submucosal myomas. Endometrial pathologies subsequently became indications for use of the resectoscope (endometrial ablation).

In endometrial resection, all or most of the endometrium is removed. The procedure is combined with the destruction of the superficial layer of the myometrium and is performed under visual guidance. Six to eight millimeters of thickness of the endometrium is resected or destroyed. This resection includes the base of the glands and the internal longitudinal layer of the myometrium, and preserves the external circular layer and its venous plexus.

ANATOMY AND PATHOPHYSIOLOGY

Anatomy of the endometrium (Figure 1).

A – Internal longitudinal layer

1 – External circular layer

B – Venous plexus

2 – Functional endometrium

To determine the edges of the resection, knowledge of the anatomy of the pelvis is essential (Figure 2).

In women of childbearing age, abnormal uterine bleeding can be linked to local or systemic abnormalities. These abnormalities can be secondary to organic pathologies of the uterine cavity, such as the presence of polyps, fibroids or endometrial hyperplasia, all of which alter the hemostatic mechanism of the endometrium. In the absence of these pathologies, uterine bleeding is defined as functional.

INDICATIONS

Hysteroscopic endometrial ablation is indicated for functional bleeding when medical therapy (progestogens, antihemorrhagic treatment, intrauterine device with levonorgestrel) fails or is contraindicated. This endoscopic procedure is only indicated for women who no longer want to become pregnant, because the mucosal destruction that is produced seriously compromises any

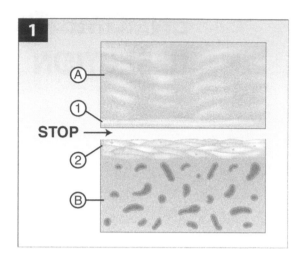

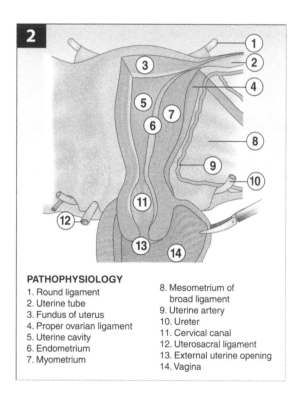

PATHOPHYSIOLOGY

1. Round ligament
2. Uterine tube
3. Fundus of uterus
4. Proper ovarian ligament
5. Uterine cavity
6. Endometrium
7. Myometrium
8. Mesometrium of broad ligament
9. Uterine artery
10. Ureter
11. Cervical canal
12. Uterosacral ligament
13. External uterine opening
14. Vagina

subsequent possibility of conception. Nevertheless, it should not be considered a permanent contraceptive procedure and patients should be advised to continue to use protective contraceptive measures.

ENDOMETRIAL RESECTION

- INDICATION: TREATMENT OF DUB
- PREOP THINNING: GNRH AGONIST
- ANESTHESIA: GENERAL OR REGIONAL
- EQUIPMENT: 12° HYSTEROSCOPE WITH INFLOW/OUTFLOW CHANNELS, DISTENSION MEDIA, FLUID MONITORING DEVICE, ELECTROSURGICAL GENERATOR
- AVERAGE TREATMENT TIME: 40+ MIN.

GOAL OF THE PROCEDURE

The goal of the procedure is to avoid a hysterectomy for a functional pathology. The resection technique is either complete with a high rate of resulting amenorrhea or hypomenorrhea, or partial with preservation of the isthmus. In the latter case, the patient's menstrual cycles are preserved. The indication for one technique over the other is more a sociological and behavioral issue than a medical one.

ENDOMETRIAL RESECTION

CONTRAINDICATIONS:

- ATYPICAL OR MALIGNANT ENDOMETRIAL LESION DETECTED DURING DIAGNOSTIC HYSTEROSCOPY AND ENDOMETRIAL BIOPSY
- A LARGE UTERUS, WHICH OFTEN LEADS TO FAILURE OF THE TECHNIQUE
- CONTRAINDICATIONS TO ANESTHESIA

PREOPERATIVE WORKUP

The preoperative workup should give a complete diagnosis of the intracavitary pathology (submucous leiomyoma, polyp) or myometrial pathology (interstitial fibroid, adenomyosis) that can account for the abnormal bleeding. It should also ensure that there is no suspicious lesion. The workup includes a pelvic (preferably endo-vaginal) ultrasonography and a diagnostic hysteroscopy with biopsy of the endometrium. The SIS or hysteroscopy may be performed in an outpatient setting before determining a surgical indication or as the first step of the surgical procedure. It verifies the regularity of the mucosa, ruling out the presence of a malignant endometrial lesion. If the findings are abnormal, a biopsy is performed and the indication is modified.

A preoperative treatment of GnRH agonists can be administered to thin down the endometrium. However, no studies have proven that this treatment improves long-term results, even though the medical preparation reduces operation time, increases efficacy of the procedure, and decreases the possibility of fluid overload. Some operators prefer to use dilute vasopressin (10 units in 50 mL saline) injected as 3 or 4 mL into the stroma of the cervix which causes intense myometrial and arterial wall contractions for 20–30 minutes.

USE OF VASOPRESSIN

- Preparation: 20 µ/100 cc saline = 0.2 µ/cc
- Direct intracervical injection at 4 and 8 o'clock
- Alert anesthesiologist
- Aspirate before injection
- Administer 10 cc/side = 4 units

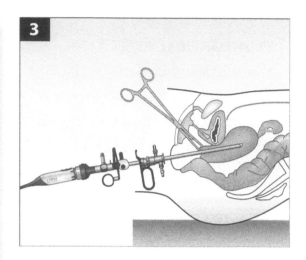

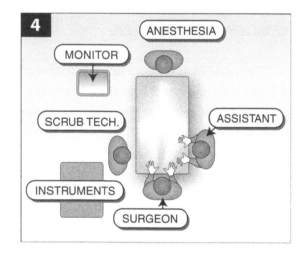

OPERATING ROOM SET-UP

PATIENT

General anesthesia, local-regional anesthesia, or paracervical block anesthesia;

Lithotomy position: legs spread at a 45° angle, thighs at a 90° angle from the surface of the table and knees bent at a 90° angle. This position allows good manipulation of the resectoscope (Figure 3);

Perineal and cervicovaginal preparation with povidone iodine;

Urinary catheter (optional). The bladder has to be emptied to optimize the uterine position for the procedure.

TEAM (The operating room set-up is presented on Figure 4)

The surgeon is seated between the patient's legs.

The assistant stands to the right of the surgeon.

The anesthesiologist is at the patient's head.

EQUIPMENT

Hysteroscopic unit and monitor

High-frequency electrosurgical generator

Instrument table

Operating table to the surgeon's right

Anesthetic unit

Equipment placed to the surgeon's left:

• Endocamera and monitor;

• Devices to control pressure and flow of distension media: a constant uterine distension must be maintained. The pressure is controlled continually by suction and irrigation pumps;

• Standard or specifically adapted tubing for each type of pump;

• Distension medium: sorbitol and glycol are the media most commonly used with monopolar cautery. With bipolar cautery, saline is used (to lower the risk of metabolic complications of fluid overload) (See Chapter 20);

• Light source: the same type of xenon light source is used for diagnostic hysteroscopy, surgical hysteroscopy, and laparoscopy;

• High frequency electrosurgical generator: unipolar electrosurgery uses high-frequency current (>300,000 Hz) (see chapter 5). Division of tissues is performed with an unmodulated current that produces a rapid rise in temperature. The unit is set to 100 W cutting current. In bipolar electrosurgery, the operating channel is 24 Fr "spray" and "desiccation" modes are available. The maximum power used by the generators is 200 W (See Chapter 20).

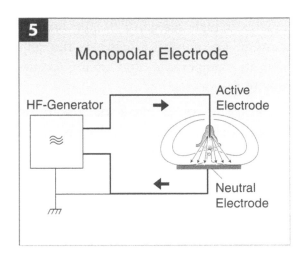

MONOPOLAR SURGERY

Current flow in monopolar surgery is from an active electrode, through tissue and returned to the generator via a large surface area plate. The high power density at the active electrode creates the desired tissue effect while the very low power density at the return electrode ensures the safe return of current (Figure 5).

BIPOLAR SURGERY

With the use of two electrodes placed close to each other, current is passed through the tissue placed between the two electrodes. This is a safer form of electrosurgery as the patient's body is not part of the electrical circuit. A special generator is used for the bipolar method (Figure 6).

On activation of bipolar energy, small steam bubbles form at the active electrode as the tip approaches the boiling point. The vapor pocket around the tip creates a high resistance to the flow of current. The generator increases the voltage to compensate and arcing occurs within the pocket.

As tissue comes into contact with the vapor pocket, the tissue forms part of the return circuit. Tissue adjacent to the vapor pocket has increased resistance due to the thermal effect of the hot saline. The current flows out of the saline and back to the return electrode, choosing the path of least resistance.

During desiccation mode, a vapor pocket does not form and tissue forms part of the return circuit. In contrast to conventional electrosurgery generators, the voltage used during coagulation is less than that used during cutting.

The voltage settings with hysteroscopic bipolar electrodes are generally less than those used in laparoscopic surgery. The generator has 3 pre-set non-modulated current settings: VC1, VC2 and VC3, two blend current settings: BL1 and BL2, and one modulated current setting: DES. Upon connecting the electrodes to the generator, the default setting is VC1, which gives maximal tissue effect. With VC2 and VC3, the vapor pocket is smaller, resulting in less tissue effect.

INSTRUMENTS

The equipment for performing the endometrial resection is presented on Figure 7.

• Hegar's dilators (No. 3 to No. 10, diameter increasing from 0.5 to 1 mm);

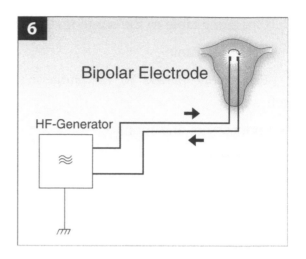

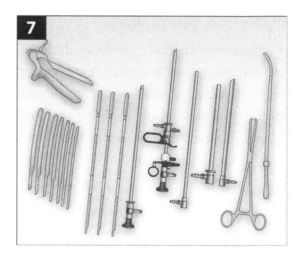

MONOPOLAR VS BIPOLAR

MONOPOLAR RESECTOSCOPE

• SORBITOL
• 4 mm, 90o LOOP ELECTRODE
• 60 TO 100 W CUTTING CURRENT

VERSAPOINT™ RESECTOSCOPE

• SALINE
• VERSAPOINT RESECTION LOOP
• 100 TO 130W VAPOR CUT

- Speculum with detachable blades;

- Resection electrode (4 mm) ending with a 90° loop-wire electrode for monopolar hysteroscopy, or a 90° 24 Fr cutting loop (2 mm) or a 5 Fr tip for bipolar hysteroscopy (Figure 8);

- Coagulation electrode: Rollerball that rotates on an axis for monopolar surgery or the 0° electrode which is 8 mm wide and ablates tissue without any residual chips;

- Rigid endoscope between 2.7 and 4 mm in diameter; the direction of view normally used in hysteroscopy is 12° wide-angle telescope;

- Resectoscope: 7 mm to 9 mm with two channels, one internal (irrigation) and one external (suction) for monopolar hysteroscopy, or 5 mm to 9 mm with two channels and a double current operation channel for bipolar hysteroscopy. In all cases it has an operative handle: passive (electrode in) or active (electrode out) (Figure 9) (See Chapter 5);

- Hysteroscope;

- Irrigation and suction channels;

- Two single-tooth tenaculum graspers;

- Uterine sound hysterometer (a sound with centimeter markings).

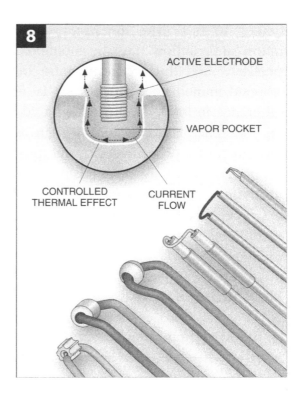

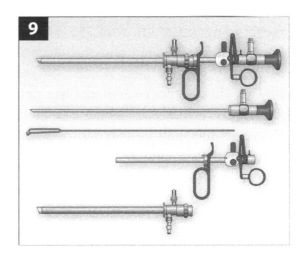

FLUID MANAGEMENT

MONOPOLAR SYSTEM

The resection techniques described use monopolar current. The suction-irrigation pump must be preset to maintain an intrauterine pressure of 100 mmHg, a 250 mL/s flow rate, a 0.2 bar suction pressure and the electrosurgical generator set at 45 W of power. The procedure must not last longer than 45 minutes. The total volume of liquid used must be

Chapter 13

166 | ENDOMETRIAL RESECTION . . . .

limited to 6 L. The distension liquid inflow and outflow must be monitored precisely, and the procedure must be stopped immediately if there is a large difference in inflow and outflow (a 700 mL difference is acceptable). If there is too much of a difference, or if the procedure lasts too long, a chemistry panel must be performed immediately after the procedure to check for a metabolic complication (hyponatremia) (See Chapter 20).

BIPOLAR SYSTEM

Bipolar spray electrosurgery is a more recent system. Its efficacy seems to be equivalent to monopolar electrosurgery, with a decrease in morbidity. The suction-irrigation pump should be preset to maintain a flow of 250 mL/s, a pressure of 80 mmHg and the electrosurgical generator set at 100 W of power. This system uses electrolyte rich fluids like saline or Ringer's lactate. However, the fluid loss should be monitored and kept under 2000 mL. There are no limits to the duration of the procedure.

> ### PREVENTIVE STRATEGIES FOR INTRAVASATION OF MEDIA
>
> - CONTROL OF INTRAUTERINE PRESSURE
> - MAINTAIN STRICT I AND O
> - AVOID EXCESSIVE OPERATING TIME

OPERATIVE TECHNIQUE

DILATION OF THE CERVIX

Bimanual examination is performed to evaluate the position of the uterus before dilation. This lowers the risk of perforation. A speculum with detachable blades is inserted and the cervix is grasped with 2 single-tooth tenacula placed in a 3 o'clock and 9 o'clock position to bring the uterus into an intermediary position. The procedure routinely begins with a diagnostic hysteroscopy if this was not done during the preoperative evaluation. The cervix is then dilated with Hegar's dilators, using progressively larger ones until a 9 mm dilator can be inserted when using a 9 mm monopolar resectoscope or 24 Fr bipolar resectoscope.

INSERTING THE RESECTOSCOPE

The endocamera, the resectoscope and the electrode are then assembled and connected to the xenon light source, the hysteroscopic unit, the electrosurgical generator and the suction-irrigation tubing. Care must be taken to remove all air bubbles from the tubing. The resectoscope is then introduced under videoscopic guidance (Figure 10).

RESECTION TECHNIQUE

The resection is usually begun on the posterior surface, creating a groove from the fundus of the uterus to the isth-

RESECTION TECHNIQUE

- REMOVE ALL BUBBLES FROM TUBING
- BEGIN ON POSTERIOR SURFACE, TRAVEL CLOCKWISE
- CAREFUL AT MARGINS OF ISTHMIC PORTION OF UTERUS, CORNUA & ENDOCERVICAL CANAL
- ONLY ACTIVATE ELECTRODE WHILE RETRACTING LOOP
- REMOVE SHAVINGS AS NEEDED
- ROLLERBALL AT END

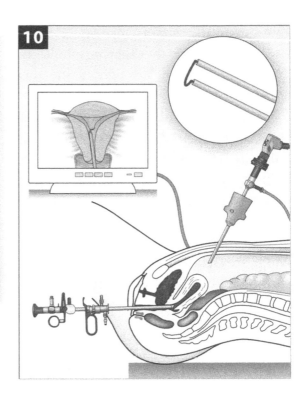

mus with a regular, continuous motion. The initial groove is used to determine how deep the resection must be, stopping on the muscular wall whose limits are defined by the external circular fibers of the myometrium, before the venous plexus layer (Figure 11). Classically, the resection of the endometrium is completed in a clockwise direction, and includes the posterior surface, the left edge, the anterior surface, and the right edge – removing the hysteroscope to empty the uterus. The margins of the isthmic portion of the uterus must be preserved due to the proximity of the uterine vessels. The endocervical portion must not be resected, to avoid endocervical adhesions that can lead to pain. In partial endometrial ablation, 1 cm of the supra-isthmic endometrial cuff is left in place. The shavings of the endometrium are collected for histologic examination using

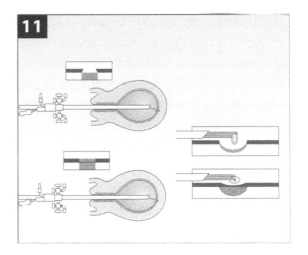

the loop or a blunt dissector. Preferably, the shavings are not removed as they are resected, but pushed towards the bottom of the cavity and removed at the end of the procedure. When endometrectomies are performed for postmenopausal patients or on a small uterus (≤6 cm), the shavings must be removed regularly throughout the procedure.

Monopolar electroendosurgery is used to perform the resection and coagulation for elective hemostasis. The bipolar electroendosurgery uses tissue vaporization and desiccation for elective hemostasis. Care must be taken not to perform aggressive resection at the cornual area and to avoid perforation also at the area of the uterine arteries.

END OF PROCEDURE

The hysteroscope is then removed and the loop resection electrode is replaced by a rollerball coagulation electrode equipped with a metal ball that rotates on an axis (Figure 12). This ensures a homogeneous coagulation. As the uterine wall is thinner at the level of the ostia, and because of the difficulty involved in resecting the fundus of the uterus, it may be easier to begin the procedure by coagulating the 2 ostia and the fundus of the uterus.

During the resection of the endometrium, hemostasis is performed as needed with elective coagulation of the vessels. At the end of the procedure, irregularities of the uterine wall must be eliminated. These irregularities are left in place until the end of the procedure to be used as anatomical landmarks.

However, if the cavity is too small to move the resectoscope, it is possible to use a 5 Fr tip for bipolar hysteroscopy.

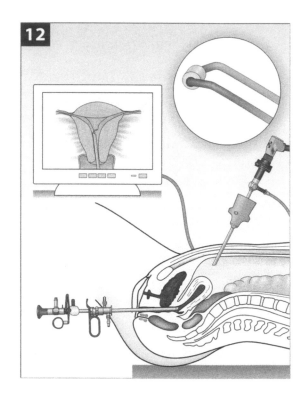

In this case, we used a spring electrode, 1.2 mm in diameter with a large surface area which makes it suitable for tissue vaporization and debulking (Figure 13).

COMPLICATIONS

MECHANICAL COMPLICATIONS

Uterine perforation may occur either during dilation of the cervix or during the resection. There is a risk of visceral burns if the perforation is not detected. To prevent perforation during dilation of the cervix, it is advisable to facilitate cervical dilation in nulliparous patients. The use of intermediary-sized Hegar's dilators (e.g., 7.5, 8.5) can also be helpful. Prevention of perforation during resection is dependent on the surgeon's compliance to certain operative rules. Constant good visualization is mandatory. In addition, it is recommended to continually extract the chips of the endometrium as they are resected, rather than push them towards the bottom of the cavity. Resection should be performed by applying energy only when the electrode is withdrawn back (Figure 14).

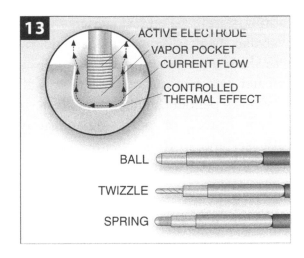

UTERINE PERFORATION WITH ACTIVATED ELECTRODE

- UTERINE PERFORATION = TERMINATION!

- MUST EVALUATE FOR VISCERAL INSULT

- CONSIDER LAPAROSCOPY OR EXPLORATORY SURGERY TO SURVEY FOR DIRECT THERMAL INSULT TO VISCERA

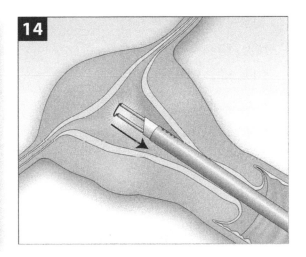

BLEEDING COMPLICATIONS

Bleeding is usually minimal and stops after a few hours. Prevention of bleeding correlates to the prevention of perforations. More serious bleeding complications may occur, and the need to resort to hysterectomy has been reported in several studies. To prevent this complication, hemostasis of the divided vessels must be carefully performed as required during the procedure. Hemostasis may be achieved with the rollerbar or the rollerball electrode that is activated against the bleeding vessel (Figure 15).

POSTOPERATIVE INFECTION

Post-hysteroscopic endometritis occurs in 1% to 5% of cases justifying the systematic use of intraoperative prophylactic antibiotics (cephalosporin). The use of preoperative antibiotics must be administered to those women with valvular heart disease, and should be considered in cases where there is a greater risk for infection, such as with insulin-dependent diabetes mellitus, a recent history of pelvic inflammatory disease, and in those women taking a high dosage of corticosteroids.

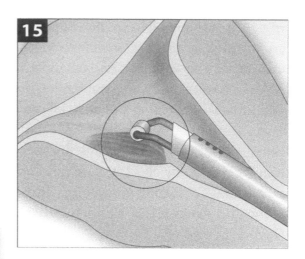

PREOPERATIVE ANTIBIOTICS?

- HIGH RISK PATIENTS
- VALVULAR DISEASE
- DIABETES MELLITUS
- PRIOR PID
- HIGH DOSE CORTICOSTEROIDS

METABOLIC COMPLICATIONS

Transurethral Resection Syndrome (TURP) (See Chapter 20) was first described by urologists. It is the result of the intravascular passage of a significant quantity of irrigation fluid, and can lead to hemodilution. This is discussed thoroughly in Chapters 3, 4 and 20.

GAS EMBOLISM

Nitrogen is principally responsible for the clinical symptomatology associated with room air embolization. To decrease this risk, the surgeon may avoid entry of air into the uterus by using a Y-shape tubing set on the fluid in-flow line in order to reduce air entrainment during bag changes; should avoid Trendelenburg position to ensure the gradient of pressure is unmodified; and should minimize the frequency of removal and reinsertion of hysteroscopic devices.

CONCLUSIONS

The development of endoscopic techniques have modified operative indications in gynecology, with a trend towards the development of conservative treatment options. In cases of abnormal uterine bleeding, medical therapy is often ineffective. Endometrial hysteroscopic resection is a rapid procedure with few intraoperative complications, provided the rules of safety are respected. The technique can be proposed for all patients who are approaching menopause and who present with a menometrorrhagia that is resistant to medical therapy. The functional results of endometrial ablation compare favorably to those of curettage. The psychological advantages of this method compared to hysterectomy are indisputable. Future developments should aim at reducing complications related to the procedure and improving its efficacy. Repeated endometrial resection is possible in cases of recurrence of dysfunctional uterine bleeding or in cases with pain and hematometra due to the obstruction of the lower parts of the uterine cavity.

Chapter 13

172 | ENDOMETRIAL RESECTION ....

SUGGESTED READING:

McCausland V, Fileds A, Townsend. Tuboovarian abscesses after operative hysteroscopy. J Reprod Med 1993;38:56

Neuwirth RS. A new technique for an additional experience with hysteroscopic resection of submucous fibroid. Am J Obstet Gynecol 1978;131:91-4

Overton C, Hargreaves J, Maresh M. A national survey of the complications of endometrial destruction for menstrual disorders: The MISTLETOE study. Br J Obstet Gynaecol 1997;104:1351-9

THERMACHOICE BALLOON ABLATION

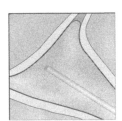

Marlies Y. Bongers, M.D., Ph.D.

The first report on the thermal ablation balloon appeared in 1994. Dr. Robert Neuwirth developed this device, initially referred to as the "endometrial ablator." GYNECARE THERMACHOICE Uterine Balloon Therapy System (Gynecare, Johnson & Johnson, NJ, USA) was the first second-generation ablation technique commercially available and has since been thoroughly evaluated.

PATIENT SELECTION

Women suffering from menorrhagia have several treatment options, including balloon endometrial ablation. Patients must have completed childbearing and be committed to using contraception consistently and correctly until menopause. In the last decade, the introduction of transvaginal sonography, saline infusion sonography, and hysteroscopy has enhanced our ability to diagnose intracavitary abnormalities. The Instructions for use (IFU) approved by the FDA, states that the "safety and effectiveness of GYNECARE THERMACHOICE UBT System has not been fully evaluated in patients with submucosal myomas . . ."One randomized clinical trial, however found that ThermaChoice was as effective as rollerball in treating women with submucosal myomas." The authors found an 89% reduction in bleeding in both arms at one year. While menorrhagia may be caused by intracavitary abnormalities, menorrhagia can also occur in women without such uterine irregularities.

When intracavitary abnormalities are not present, women suffering from menorrhagia are said to have dysfunctional uterine bleeding. Dysfunctional uterine bleeding is defined as periodic uterine blood loss in excess of 80 mL per cycle occurring in the absence of structural uterine disease. GYNECARE THERMACHOICE Uterine Balloon Therapy System balloon ablation for women with dysfunctional uterine bleeding is discussed in this chapter.

THERMACHOICE EMBA

- INDICATION: TREATMENT OF DUB IN UTERI 4–10CM, SMALL TRIAL – POSSIBLE USE WITH SUBMUCOUS FIBROID
- PREOP THINNING: CURETTAGE, GNRH AGONIST
- ANESTHESIA: GENERAL, REGIONAL OR LOCAL
- EQUIPMENT: THERMACHOICE DISPOSABLE KIT & GENERATOR, 30CC SYRINGE, DEXTROSE 5%, SPECULUM, TENACULUM, UTERINE SOUND
- AVERAGE TREATMENT TIME: 10 MIN

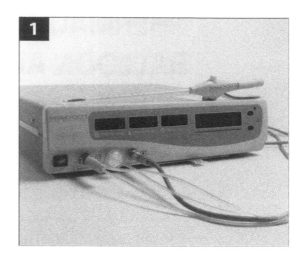

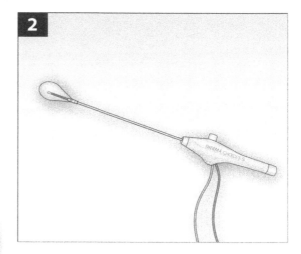

TECHNIQUE

The ThermaChoice balloon ablation system is currently in its third generation. The device consists of a generator (Figure 1) and a silicone balloon catheter (Figure 2) with an outer diameter of 5 mm. A plastic catheter connects the silicone balloon to three lines: one for electrical connection, one for an impeller cable, and the other for liquid. The silicone balloon conforms to the uterine cavity at relatively low pressures but is optimized to operate at an intrauterine pressure of approximately 170 mmHg. The balloon is filled with 5% dextrose in water by a syringe. The distal end of the catheter forms the center axis of the balloon, inside of which there is a heating element, two thermistors (surrounded by a perforated heat shield), and an impeller (Figure 3). The thermistors monitor the temperature of the fluid within the balloon. The heating element regulates the temperature of the fluid to 87°C (170° F) during an 8-minute treatment cycle with pressure being maintained at 150–200 mmHg. The impeller circulates the heated fluid to ensure that it is distributed evenly throughout the balloon.

The generator controls temperature and time and monitors pressure. First the unit records the instantaneous pressure in the catheter. If the pressure is outside the 45–200 mmHg range the heating unit shuts down. The heat control measures the instantaneous temperature within the balloon and provides 12-V direct-current electricity for the heating coil located in the perforated heat shield at the center of the balloon. The heating unit is limited to 92° C. If the temperature exceeds this limit, the heating element will switch off automatically. The third control function is operating time. The control unit has a digital clock for recording elapsed time of treatment. After a preheating period to obtain a temperature of 87° C, the gen-

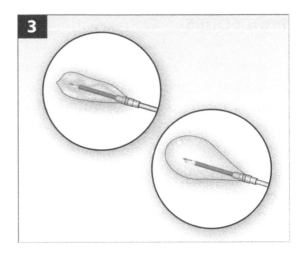

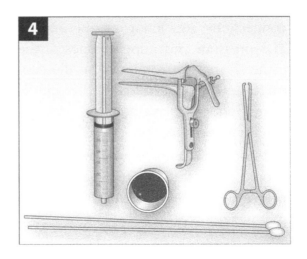

erator will then heat for 8 minutes before automatically turning off.

Previous generations of the GYNECARE THERMACHOICE Uterine Balloon Therapy System are being phased out. The first generation utilized a latex balloon. ThermaChoice II switched to a silicone balloon and added the impeller. The catheter used in the currently marketed version retains the impeller and uses a more compliant silicone balloon.

PROCEDURE

Instruments needed to initiate the procedure include: a speculum, a tenaculum, a uterine sound, a 60cc syringe, dextrose 5%, and a ThermaChoice balloon catheter (Figure 4).

The Controller unit is connected to the power supply and to the umbilical cord that connects it to the balloon catheter. The catheter is taken out of the sterile package and connected to the umbilical cord by matching the colored connections and lining up the arrows. The pressure and impeller lines of the catheter are also connected to the controller unit. When the controller unit is turned on it displays numbers for pressure, temperature, and clock displays.

Prior to starting the procedure, one should prime the catheter and titrate the pressures in the balloon by doing the following:

• Fill syringe with 15cc D5W. Expel extra air.

• Keep catheter in vertical position with balloon facing the floor. (Keep in this position until priming is complete.)

• Attach syringe to top of catheter.

• Press trumpet valve and SLOWLY inject 10cc D5W into balloon to demonstrate no leakage.

• With balloon still in vertical position, press trumpet valve and withdraw all air and fluid until the controller shows negative pressure between 150–200 mmHg (Figure 5).

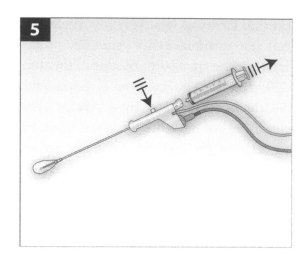

5

THERMACHOICE TECHNIQUE

• EASY TO USE & ASSEMBLE (INSTRUCTION CARD)

• PRIME CATHETER (15CC D5W) & TITRATE PRESSURES IN BALLOON TO −150 TO −200 MMHG

• BALLOON CATHETER IS PLACED IN UTERINE CAVITY

• BALLOON FILLED WITH D5W TO 160–180 MMHG

• MAX OF 30CC OF FLUID

• FLUID PREHEATED TO 87° C (<1MIN), ABLATION X 8MIN, COOLING (<1MIN)

After the above is completed, the procedure may be performed safely. Steps involved in performing the ablation are as follows:

• With the patient in lithotomy position, the speculum is introduced and the cervix is grasped with a tenaculum;

• A paracervical block using a long acting local anesthetic (along with pre-operative administration of NSAIDS) can help reduce post-operative pain;

• The depth of the uterine cavity should be measured (Figure 6), after which the balloon catheter is introduced, usually without dilating the cervix. The 5 mm outer diameter makes this introduction easy;

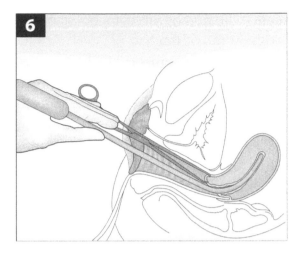

• After insertion of the balloon catheter into the uterine cavity, the balloon is filled with dextrose 5% until a maximum pressure of 160–180 mmHg is reached (Figure 7). This usually requires 10–30cc of dextrose to reach the desired pressure. Add fluid as necessary (up to 30 mL) to titrate the pressure. The valve control button on the catheter must be pressed in order to inject or remove fluid from the balloon (Figure 8). As fluid is injected into the balloon, the uterus will relax causing the pressure within the balloon to decline. One should then refill the catheter carefully and wait until the pressure stabilizes between 160–180 mmHg. Over-zealous filling of the balloon to pressures over 220 mmHg will result in bursting of the safety valve thus making the balloon unusable. Allow the pressure to stabilize to 160–200 mmHg for 30–45 seconds before pressing the start button. If pressure cannot be stabilized with 30 mL of fluid, check for uterine perforation and/or balloon catheter leak. This is an important safety feature of the device. If the catheter has perforated and the balloon is extrauterine, the pres-

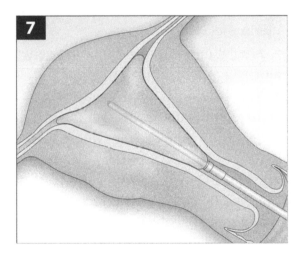

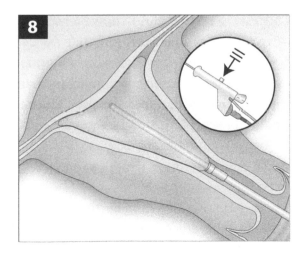

sure will not be able to be stabilized with 30 mL of fluid;

• After the pressure in the balloon has stabilized, pressing the start button will begin the preheating process. The preheating process may take up to 4 minutes, but it is usually 15–45 seconds. Hold the catheter immobile in the center of the uterine cavity during the treatment cycle and be ready to tell jokes for 8 minutes. At a temperature of 87° C the 8-minute treatment will begin. During the treatment cycle a fall in intrauterine pressure is frequently observed due to uterine relaxation;

• After 8 minutes of heating the generator will automatically switch off;

• The balloon is then emptied with a syringe and withdrawn from the uterus.

Figure 9 shows the hysteroscopic view of the endometrium before and after the ablation procedure. The ThermaChoice balloon is recommended for endometrial ablation with the uterine size sounding up to 12 cm in length although in the United States it is indicated for uteri that sound between 4 and 10 cm. The machine, however, is not capable of preheating more than 60cc of dextrose fluid to the recommended ablation temperature. The machine cannot be overridden and the procedure in patients with large uterine cavities may have to be abandoned.

If during the ablation procedure a drop in intrauterine pressure is experienced below 140 mmHg, the manufacturer of the device does not recommend

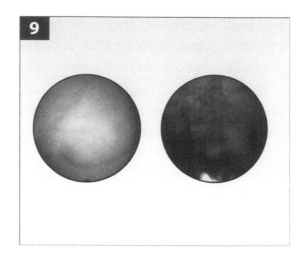

adding additional fluid to the balloon to elevate the pressure. This is due to the concern that additional fluid may decrease the ablation process, and that a precipitous drop in pressure may reflect a balloon leak or a perforation. Although in practice, addition of more fluid, if done carefully, will not hamper the ablation procedure.

The balloon procedure may be performed under general anesthesia, regional anesthesia by a spinal block, or local anesthesia. Pure local anesthesia consists of a paracervical block. The lack of need for cervical dilation is an important advantage for balloon ablation in an outpatient setting. However, painless ablation under local anesthesia is hampered due to the nerve innervation of the fundus uteri from thoracal 12th segment, which is not blocked by paracervical anesthesia. A painless outpatient procedure with balloon ablation can be supported by intravenous sedation. However, intravenous sedation in an outpatient clinic requires an infra-structure which includes electrocardiac monitoring, pulsoximetry monitoring, and anesthesiologist support to perform this minor surgery safely. Nevertheless, the outpatient approach as opposed to operating room expense is more cost effective. Also, specially trained staff is not necessary for balloon ablation pro-cedures.

EFFECTIVENESS

GYNECARE THERMACHOICE™ Uter-ine Balloon Therapy System has been compared to rollerball ablation in a ran-domized controlled trial. Results have been reported at 1, 2, 3, and 5 years after treatment. The GYNECARE THER-MACHOICE™ Uterine Balloon Therapy System balloon ablation is the only sec-ond-generation ablation device in which long-term follow-up results have been reported. The results of the RCT are presented in Table 1. At 3 and 5-years follow-up, both patient satisfac-tion and the hysterectomy rate (30%) are comparable between treatment modalities, with the amenorrhea rate being somewhat lower in the balloon group (Table 1). Note that the hysterec-tomy rate includes hysterectomy for all indications, not exclusively menorrha-gia. These results are consistent with the findings in several non-randomized studies in which GYNECARE THERMA-CHOICE™ Uterine Balloon Therapy System is compared to TCRE, as well as

with the findings in various prospective observational studies.

The lower amenorrhea rate after bal-loon ablation was the motivation in studying optimal heating time. The effectiveness of 8 versus 16 minutes of heating in the treatment of menorrhagia with hot fluid balloon ablation was compared. Failure rates of the hot fluid balloon therapy, defined as either hys-terectomy or dissatisfaction with the treatment result, were not significantly different in the two treatment groups (Hazard Rate Ratio 1.0; 95% confidence interval 0.93 to 1.2). This study demon-strated no advantage to doubling the heating period of the balloon ablation therapy from 8 to 16 minutes. The sup-ply of energy to the endometrium is likely balanced with the removal of this energy by uterine blood vessels. However, balloon pressures greater than 150 mmHg did increase the effective-ness of the treatment. At higher pres-sures (150–180 mmHg) the endometri-um is flattened and thinned out, and tighter balloon contact with the uterine wall may allow for greater local thermal injury and a higher degree of endomy-ometrial coagulation.

Pretreatment of the endometrium can be performed with GnRH analogues or with suction curettage. This is done to decrease the thickness of the endome-trial layer prior to ablative treatment. Whether pre-operative thinning of the endometrium with GnRH analogues will improve the success rate of balloon ablation is still a matter of debate. Although, statistically higher rates of post procedure amenorrhea in women who received pre-operative depot GnRH agonist have been reported, it did not improve treatment outcome in terms of the need for surgical re-intervention. Endometrial thickness of more than 4 mm, however, is associated with an unfavorable prognostication and GnRH pre-treatment may be advantageous to diminish the endometrial layer.

THERMACHOICE RESULTS

- Max tissue necrosis: 0.33 mm mid-body, 0.95 mm fundus

- 95% reported normal bleeding or less without additional intervention at 5yrs

- At 3–5yrs: 11–24% amenorrhea rate, 64–93% satisfaction rate

CONCERNS

Serious complications of GYNECARE THERMACHOICE™ Uterine Balloon Therapy System ablation are extremely uncommon. In every day use it is a very simple and safe ablation procedure.

ThermaChoice™ ablation is not contraceptive; therefore, another form of contraception is necessary to prevent pregnancy. Pregnancy after balloon ablation is considered a complication. Pregnancy is estimated to occur in 0.2% to 1.6% of all endometrial ablation cases. Such pregnancies have an increased risk of pregnancy loss, as well as other obstetric complications. A possible explanation for these complications is the sub-optimal and/or abnormal attachment of placental tissue to the denuded endometrium.

The potential delay of diagnosing endometrial cancer is a disadvantage of all endometrial ablation techniques. A majority of cases of endometrial cancer diagnosed after endometrial ablation were preceded by a pretreatment endometrial biopsy containing atypical hyperplasia. Thus, it is important to take an accurate endometrial sampling before ablation treatment. The ablation procedure should not be performed if the biopsy contains (pre) malignant tissue. Also, endometrial ablation should not be offered for the treatment of abnormal uterine bleeding due to endometrial hyperplasia. This is especially of concern in patients with diabetes, extreme obesity, or hypertension. While these co-morbidities increase the risk of major surgery, thus making less invasive procedures more attractive, these patients are at an increased risk for endometrial cancer. Despite the existence of endometrial ablations with first generation devices for more than twenty years, it is still unclear to what extent endometrial ablation may delay the diagnosis of endometrial cancer.

PROGNOSTIC VALUES

Potential prognostic factors for assessing the success of balloon ablation were evaluated in two trials. In the French study, a retroverted uterus was associated with an increased failure rate (Hazard Rate Ratio 3.9; 95% CI 1.2 13). Predictive factors for adverse outcome in the Dutch study were a retroverted uterus (Hazard Rate Ratio 3.3; 95% CI 1.2 to 8.6), pretreatment endometrial thickness of at least 4 mm (Hazard Rate Ratio 3.6; 95% CI 1.3 to 11), and the duration of menstruation (Hazard Rate Ratio 1.2; 95% CI 1.0 to 1.3, per day in excess of 9 days). The risk of an adverse outcome declined steadily with increasing age Hazard Rate Ratio 0.86; 95% CI 0.77 to 0.96, per year over 42 years of age). Uterine depth and dysmenorrhea were not predictive factors affecting outcome. The relative unfavorable outcome with a retroverted uterus may be due to the anterior position of the heater element inside the balloon.

CONCLUSION

ThermaChoice™ endometrial ablation is a simple, safe, and effective ablation method. Long-term follow-up results from a randomized controlled trial show that after 5 years 70% of the patients did not need a hysterectomy.

SUGGESTED READING:

Neuwirth RS, Duran A, Singer A, MacDonald R, Bolduc L. The endometrial ablator: a new instrument. Obstet Gynecol 1994;83:792-796

Singer A, Almanza R, Guttierez G, Haber G, Bolduc LR, Neuwirth R. Preliminary clinical experience with a thermal balloon endometrial ablation method to treat menorrhagia. Obstet Gynecol 1994;83:732-734

Vilos GA, Vilos EC, Pendley L. Endometrial ablation with a thermal balloon for the treatment of menorrhagia. J Am Assoc Gynecol Laparosc 1996;3:383-387

Fernandez H, Capella S, Audibert F. Uterine thermal balloon therapy under local anesthesia for the treatment of menorrhagia: a pilot study. Hum Reprod 1997;12:2511-2514

Byrd LM, Chia KV. Balloon ablation: is this an outpatient procedure? J Obstet Gynecol 2002;22:205-208

Lok I H, Chan M, Tam W H, Leung P L, Yuen P M. Patient-controlled sedation for outpatient thermal balloon endometrial ablation. J Am Assoc Gynecol Laparosc 2002;9:436-441

Meyer WR, Walsh BW, Grainger DA, Peacock LM, Loffer FD, Steege JF. Thermal balloon and rollerball ablation to treat menorrhagia: A multi-center comparison. Obstet Gynecol 1998;92:98-103

Grainger D, Tjaden B. Thermal balloon and rollerball ablation to treat menorrhagia: Two-year results from a multicenter prospective, randomized clinical trial. J Am Assoc Gynecol Laparosc 2000;7:175-179

Loffer FD. Three-year comparison of thermal balloon and rollerball ablation in treatment of menorrhagia. J Am Assoc Gynecol Laparosc 2001;8:48-54

Loffer FD Grainger D. Five-year follow-up of patients participating in a randomized trial of uterine balloon therapy versus rollerball ablation for treatment of menorrhagia. J Am Assoc Gynecol Laparosc 2002;9:429-435

Bongers MY, Mol BWJ, Brölmann HAM. Comparison of 8 versus 16 minutes heating in the treatment of menorrhagia with hot fluid balloon ablation. J Gynecol Surg 1999;15:143-147

Bongers MY, Mol BWJ, Dijkhuizen FPHLJ, Brölmann HAM. Is balloon-ablation as effective as endometrial electro-resection in the treatment of menorrhagia? J Lap Adv Surg Techn. 2000;10:85-92

Gervaise A, Fernandez H, Capella-Allouc S, Taylor S, La Vieille S, Hamou J, et al. Thermal balloon ablation versus endometrial resection for the treatment of abnormal uterine bleeding. Hum Reprod 1999;14:2743-2747

Bongers MY, Mol BWJ, Brölmann HAM. Prognostic factors for the success of thermal balloon ablation in the treatment of menorrhagia. Obstet Gynecol 2002;99:1060-1066

Amso NN, Stabinsky SA, McFaul P, Blanc B, Pendley L, Neuwirth R. Uterine thermal balloon therapy for the treatment of menorrhagia: the first 300 patients from a multi-center study. Br J Obstet Gynaecol 1998;105:517-523

HYDROTHERMAL ABLATION (HTA®)

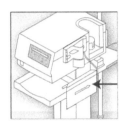

Milton H. Goldrath, M.D.

Hydro thermablation is a technique to ablate the endometrial layer of the uterus utilizing heated saline (80–90°C) introduced into the uterine cavity by a hysteroscopic system. This system is called the Hydro Thermablator® (HTA®).

Hydro thermablation is safe, simple, very effective and exceptionally easy to perform as a minor operative procedure for the treatment of menorrhagia. Since the HTA® system offers the opportunity for office-based, or ambulatory interventions, it is an attractive choice compared with traditional rollerball or resectoscopic surgery. It eliminates electrosurgical hazards and serious fluid management problems. In contrast to other "global" ablation techniques, the HTA® system offers the safety and confidence of hysteroscopic visualization throughout the procedure. It is essentially insensitive to variations from the norm regarding cavity size and shape that limit treatment devices with set sizes or shapes.

PATIENT SELECTION

Before considering endometrial ablation as a treatment for menorrhagia, uterine neoplasm must be ruled out. Depending on the age of the patient and her risk factors, this may be done with pelvic ultrasonography, saline infusion sonohysterography, or office hysteroscopy with endometrial biopsy (my personal preference). Diagnostic hysteroscopy offers a visually guided biopsy of suspicious areas that may be missed by blind biopsy, or go unrecognized by sonographic techniques. Alternatively, in low-risk patients, a small caliber suction biopsy can be performed as a "blind" procedure with the confidence that endometrial ablation with the Hydro ThermAblator® provides a "last minute" hysteroscopic look prior to treatment.

Although pharmaceuticals are highly successful in the treatment of menorrhagia due to benign causes, they are ineffective in some women. However, many women find it difficult to adhere to this form of therapy for long periods of time due to drug-related side effects. For these patients, endometrial ablation becomes an attractive alternative to hysterectomy. A history of dysmenorrhea may suggest adenomyosis as a diagnosis, and the patient should be advised that endometrial ablation may fail to provide complete relief of symptoms.

INCLUSION / EXCLUSION CRITERIA

Patients who are in good general health and who do not desire future pregnancies are good candidates for treatment with the HTA® system. Patients who present with fibroids can be treated provided the fibroids do not obscure visualization of both cornua nor distort the cavity to the extent that it prevents free circulation of fluid. Asymmetrically shaped and "T" shaped uterine cavities can be effectively treated with the circulating, heated saline of the HTA® system.

Patients should be excluded from treatment with the HTA® if they have abnormal cervical cytology, abnormal endometrial pathology or large (> 4 cm) fibroids and polyps. Patients that have had previous uterine surgeries, such as full thickness myomectomy, classic cesarean section, (except for low transverse cesarean section) uterine reconstruction or any surgery in which thinning of the myometrium could occur, should be fully evaluated before treatment with the HTA® system. Any patient who has clotting or bleeding disorders that have not been fully evaluated should not be treated. Any patient with a complete septate or bicornuate uterus should be excluded. However, patients with partial septa have been successfully treated using the HTA®. Patients who have had a low uterine cesarean section can be treated with HTA® but care should be taken to avoid perforation on dilatation.

INDICATION: HYDRO THERMABLATOR (HTA)

- TREATMENT OF DUB, BUT FIBROIDS/POLYPS AND ASYMMETRICAL CAVITY OK

- PREOP THINNING RECOMMENDED: GNRH AGONIST, OCPs, SUCTION D&C

- ANESTHESIA: GENERAL, REGIONAL, IV WITH PARACERVICAL

- EQUIPMENT: 30° OR 12° – 3 MM HYSTEROSCOPE, HTA DISPOSABLE KIT, 3 L BAG NS, HEATER CANISTER, CERVICAL SEALING TENACULUM

- AVERAGE TREATMENT TIME: 15 MIN

ENDOMETRIAL PREPARATION

Historically, optimal endometrial ablation occurs when the procedure is performed in a uterine cavity with a thin endometrium. Therefore, endometrial thinning should take place prior to the HTA® treatment in order to aid visualization and to achieve the optimum heat penetration through the endometrium into the myometrium. Ideally, the endometrium should measure < 4 mm at the time of treatment.

Endometrial thinning has been successfully accomplished prior to the HTA® procedure by means of a single injection of GnRH agonist (i.e., Lupron Depot, (Tap Pharmaceuticals, Lake Forest, IL.,) 3.75 mg IM or Zoladex, (Astrazeneca Pharmaceuticals, Inc., Wilmington, DE.,) 3.6 mg IM) with treatment being performed 21–28 days later. Danocrine, (Sanofi-Synthelabo Inc., New York.,) 400 mg BID for 25 days prior to the scheduled surgery date has been used, but patient compliance is difficult to assure due to known side effects. Another simple method is the use of continuous low-dose oral contraceptives for 1–2 cycles, with treatment scheduled for 5–8 days after withdrawal to cause a menstrual bleed and sloughing of tissue. Another option that may be considered is suction-only curettage to remove endometrial tissue and any blood or clots from the uterine cavity, rather than repeated insertions of a mechanical curette that can traumatize and over dilate the cervical canal. However, this technique is known to provide uneven thinning and can result in increased bleeding within the uterine cavity and may require extended flushing hysteroscopy to obtain clear visualization before therapy.

Patients should be instructed to discontinue use of any other hormonal medications while receiving the described hormonal agents. Patients can become pregnant during administration of the pre-treatment GnRH agonists and must be instructed to use barrier contraceptive methods. A pregnancy test should be performed on the day scheduled for endometrial ablation.

CHOICE OF SETTING

Physicians wishing to perform procedures with the HTA® system in an office setting should be experienced in the management of patient discomfort from intrauterine procedures in this setting. The facility should have the appropriate personnel and equipment to manage an unforeseen complication. Local and government regulations should be closely followed regarding surgical procedures performed in an office setting. If electing to perform an HTA® procedure without the support of general anesthesia, the physician must thoroughly evaluate the patient's psyche and anatomy so as to individually tailor pre-procedure and intra-procedure pain management. Patients with a narrow vaginal introitus, a markedly retroverted uterus or a narrow or stenotic cervix may not be ideally suited for an office-based procedure.

Many physicians choose to administer pain medication and/or anti-inflammatory medications from 24 hours to 30 minutes before the HTA® procedure. Various pre-medications, including oral Cataflam, (Novartis Pharmaceuticals Corp, East Hanover, NJ.,) oral Bextra (Pfizer, New York, NY) or Indocin, (Merck & Co., Inc. West Point, PA.,) as a rectal suppository have been utilized by physicians experienced in performing endometrial ablation with minimal anesthesia. Another very effective medication is Toradol (Roche Pharmaceuticals,

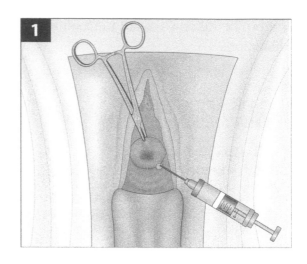

Nutley, NJ.,) 30 mg IM given about 30 minutes prior to the procedure. Atropine 0.2 mg can be given to reduce the occurrence of a vasovagal reaction.

The real key to patient comfort is the administration of an effective paracervical block, using a medication like carbocaine 1.0% without epinephrine. The volume should be limited to less than 20 cc, with 1–2 cc administered at the anterior cervical lip (prior to grasping the cervix with tenaculum), and the balance divided between 4 o'clock and 8 o'clock, taking care to avoid intra-vascular injection (Figure 1). Rather than immediately proceeding with cervical dilatation, the local anesthetic agent should be given 5–10 minutes to become effective. This time can be used to prepare the HTA® hysteroscopic sheath and camera system.

For most patients, the low-pressure distention of the uterine cavity utilized by the HTA® system is easily tolerated since the uterus is insensitive to heat, but very sensitive to increased pressure. Uterine muscle spasm and cramping are known to be caused by the considerably higher distention pressures used in other methods.

Patient complaints of intra-procedural pain will be significantly reduced when the patient has been fully informed regarding the components and the length of time required for the procedure. An ongoing dialogue characterized by warmth and empathy will dramatically lessen complaints of intra-procedural discomfort. Having the patient "participate" by viewing the video monitor throughout the procedure can also have an analgesic-like effect. If a patient has significant intra-procedure discomfort, such agents as IV Versed, (Roche Pharmaceuticals, Inc., Nutley, NJ.) IV Fentanyl, or IV Demerol, (Synofi-Synthelabo, Inc., New York, NY.,) can be used as required to provide relief.

The system and procedure is so designed that prior to treatment the uterus is inspected hysteroscopically using unheated saline solution to observe the uterine cavity and to flush out any blood that may be present due to the dilation. After the surgeon is satisfied with the appearance of the endometrium and the position of the sheath, the fluid takes approximately three minutes to heat to ablation temperature. During that time, any leakage would be readily determined by the fluid loss monitoring system. Any

loss greater than 10 cc automatically interrupts flow of fluid to the patient.

SUPPLIES AND ANCILLARY MATERIALS

- Disposable HTA® procedure kit and a spare 3 mm hysteroscope telescope with appropriate sheath adapter

- Bag of 3 liters of 0.9% normal saline

- Sterilized heater canister and a spare

- Appropriate cervical sealing tenaculum

HTA® SYSTEM PREPARATION

The HTA® System control unit can be prepared for use before the patient is in the room. This part of the procedure is performed by the operating room personnel.

Prior to use of the HTA® system, a heater canister and a spare must be properly cleaned and steam sterilized with the components disassembled. Before assembly, it must be confirmed that the base and the top of the heater canister have "O" rings properly positioned. The inner cylinder is positioned over the "O" ring in the base and then the outer protective cylinder is installed. The top contains the temperature sensing thermocouples and should be handled carefully. After aligning the top over the two cylinders, it is threaded onto the heater rod until the resistance of the "O" ring is felt. A small amount of additional tightening is required for a good seal. It is important to realize that the outer cylinder does remain loose since it plays no part in sealing in liquid (Figure 2).

When the HTA® power system is turned on, the front panel display will become illuminated and the unit will proceed through a series of self-diagnostic steps. The front panel display will guide the user step-by-step. The display will also indicate self-diagnostic messages, warnings and corrective action required if necessary. The first message prompts the user to install the heater canister and connect the thermocouple cable. The sterile heater canister is installed with the marker on its base aligned with the slot in the receptacle on the rear of the unit (Figure 3), and then the thermocouple cable is installed on the canister. The user can press start to confirm that the cable is properly connected and the thermocouples are functioning properly. Pressing start again will cause the HTA® to proceed to the next step in the setup procedure. The procedure kit contains a pictorial of the steps for installation.

Installation of the cassette, tubing and reservoir assembly is simplified if the reservoir is first installed on the unit's IV pole. The alignment pin on the base of

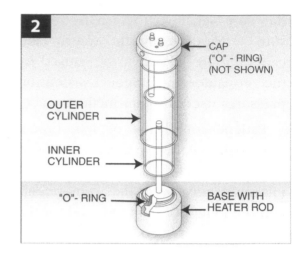

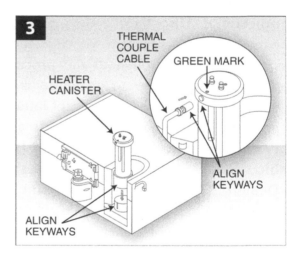

STERILE PACKAGE CONTAINS

- CONTINUOUS FLOW SHEET AND ITS INSULATED CONNECTING TUBING
- DRAIN BAG FOR COLLECTION OF FLUID
- THE FLOW CONTROLLED CASSETTE WITH TUBING AND LEVEL SENSING RESERVOIR PRE-CONNECTED
- THE PACKAGE CONTAINING THE HYSTEROSCOPE SHEATH SHOULD BE LAID ASIDE FOR LATER USE

the reservoir should be inserted in the corresponding hole in the metal lower reservoir holder. With this pin in place, the top of the reservoir with its five electronic pins can be aligned with and inserted into the multi-pin receptacle on the pole (Figure 4).

The position of the tubing within the flow-control cassette should be checked before installation to confirm that it is properly centered between the two tubing guides. The tubing must be centered to insure proper pump function. Alignment of the cassette slots located at the rear edge of the cassette with the metal tabs allows the rear edge of the cassette to be engaged on the controller unit (Figure 5). The electronic cassette latch located at the front of flow-control cassette is only open for a short time before it automatically engages. If this happens, it will be necessary to press the cassette latch release button on the front panel to allow proper and complete installation of the cassette. With the electronic latch open, the cassette can be fully installed and the mechanical latch can be closed to secure the cassette. When it is certain that the cassette is properly installed, the user can press the start button to proceed. The tubes are connected to the heater canister with the red band corresponding to the luer-lock fitting with the red marker. Following the prompt instructions, the saline bag is spiked and the clamp on the tubing is open. Continuing to follow the prompts, the IV pole is raised so that the mid-point

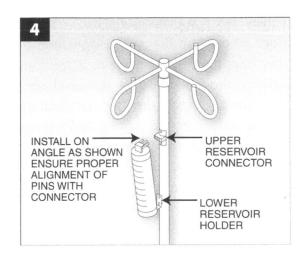

INSTALL ON ANGLE AS SHOWN ENSURE PROPER ALIGNMENT OF PINS WITH CONNECTOR

UPPER RESERVOIR CONNECTOR

LOWER RESERVOIR HOLDER

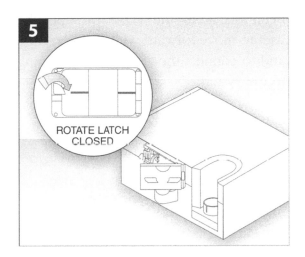

ROTATE LATCH CLOSED

of the reservoir is at a height of 115 cm above the expected position of the uterus (Figure 6). Following the prompts, the next step is to install the drain collection bag and connect its tube (Figure 7). Now, when the start button is pressed the pump begins to operate and the system begins to fill with saline, flushing air from the system. During the filling phase, the HTA® performs multiple checks of the fluid level sensors in the reservoir by opening and closing control valves in a specific sequence. This is done to confirm the proper operation of this important safety system. After confirming the operation of the level sensors, the HTA® will raise the temperature of the saline in the system from room temperature to body temperature. This confirms operation of the heater and the double temperature measurement thermocouples in the heater canister. The HTA® will only proceed if this system is properly functioning. Now that the fluid level sensors and the heating system has been checked, the HTA® prompts the user to move forward with the procedure and to connect the sheath and its tubing to the system.

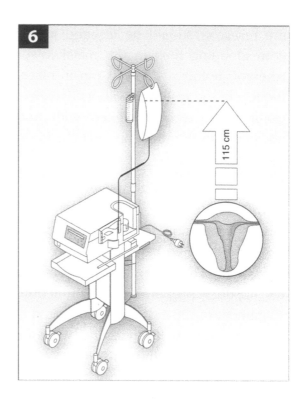

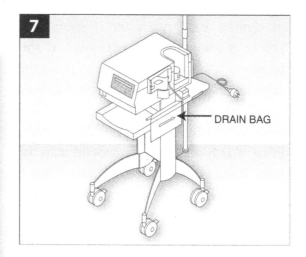

HTA SYSTEM: FUNCTION

- PROPER ASSEMBLY OF SYSTEM

- FLUID: 0.9% NS – PLACE 115CM ABOVE UTERUS

- HTA SYSTEM CHECK: FLUID LEVEL SENSORS, CONNECTIONS AND HEATING SYSTEM

- DILATE CERVIX TO 24 FR

- DIAGNOSTIC HYSTEROSCOPY X 2MIN

- TIP OF SHEATH JUST INSIDE INTERNAL OSTIUM

- HEAT 80–90° C X 3MIN, ABLATION UNDER DIRECT VISUALIZATION X 10 MIN, COOLING X 1 MIN

PATIENT PREPARATION

For the HTA® procedure, the patient is placed in the dorsdithotomy position, and then prepped and draped in the usual manner. An open-sided vaginal speculum is placed to expose the cervix and a paracervical block is administered as described previously. The HTA® hysteroscopic sheath can be prepared while the anesthetic agent is taking effect.

The HTA® hysteroscopic sheath is removed from its sterile peel-pouch and the hysteroscope of choice is connected to the sheath using an appropriate bridge or adapter (Figure 8). Such adapters are available for hysteroscope telescopes from the major manufacturers. The only requirement is that the telescope be no larger than 3 mm O.D. so that flow through the sheath is not restricted. Telescope field of view can be 0°, 12° or 30°, but the 12° version seems to be most convenient. If a 30° telescope is used, care must be taken to avoid aiming the end of the sheath at the wall of the uterine cavity if the hysteroscopic view has the tubal ostia in the 3 and 9 o'clock positions. Instead, with a 30° telescope the view of the tubal ostia should be offset from the mid position to assure that the axis of the HTA® sheath is positioned mid-cavity.

A small silicone tip is packaged with the HTA® sheath that is critical in set-up of the apparatus. It is placed over the distal end of the sheath to create a closed loop for fluid circulation (Figure 9). The Patient Sheath inflow and outflow tubes are passed from the sterile field to an assistant who removes the protective caps from the color-coded tube connectors. The assistant attaches them to the respective color coded tub-

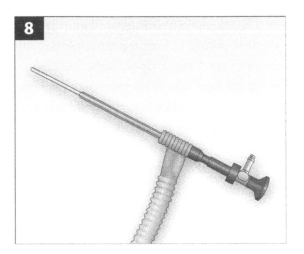

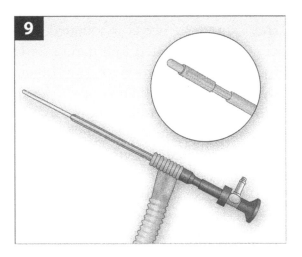

ing connections on the pump cassette (male and female luer style, purple to purple and yellow to yellow) and confirms that the flexible tip is properly and securely attached to the distal end of the HTA® sheath before pressing the "Start" button. When the start button is pushed, saline circulates through the sheath and its connecting tubes, flushing air from the system. This flushing cycle requires approximately one minute and the control unit display provides a countdown of the time remaining until completion of this cycle. During this phase, the camera and fiber optic light guide may be attached to the hysteroscopic telescope and a check for any loose connections and potential fluid leaks should be made. Particular attention should be given to the hysteroscopic telescope and adapter connection to the insulated sheath, and to the connections at the heater canister on the control unit.

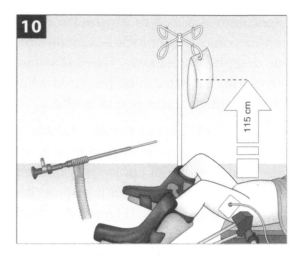

After the local anesthetic has taken effect, a tenaculum is placed at 12 o'clock and the cervix is sounded. The cervix is then dilated to 8 mm or 24 Fr. to allow the insertion of the 7.8-mm outer diameter hysteroscopic sheath. One must not overdilate the cervix. All types of hydrophilic dilators (laminaria) must be avoided since these can overdilate the cervix and prevent a good seal of the cervix around the sheath. Before proceeding, it is very important to confirm the height of the fluid reservoir on the control unit's IV pole. Be certain that the height of the IV pole is adjusted so that the mid point of the fluid reservoir ("80" mark) is no more than 115 cm (45 inches) above the patient's uterus (Figure 10). This assures that the intrauterine pressure will be 50–55 mmHg; (below the known minimum tubal opening pressure of 70 mmHg). The maximum intrauterine pressure during HTA® treatment is strictly a function of the height of the reservoir since the peristaltic pump on the HTA® control unit is an aspiration pump, the sole

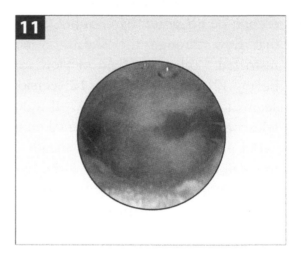

function of which is to return fluid from the uterus to the reservoir and then the heater canister for re-heating. The length of the disposable tubing set has been designed to prevent excessive elevation of the fluid reservoir.

The HTA® sheath should be gently inserted through the cervical canal into the lower uterine segment. Introduction under direct hysteroscopic visualization with saline flowing will aid in following the direction of the cervical canal. If difficulty is encountered with the insertion of the sheath, the cervix may be further dilated, however, over-dilation must be avoided in order to assure a snug fit and a good fluid seal of the cervix around the sheath during the therapy cycle.

Diagnostic hysteroscopy is performed using room temperature saline to flush the uterus. Visualization of the tubal ostia provides confirmation that the HTA® sheath has been positioned within the uterine cavity, rather than in a false passage or through a perforation (Figure 11). This examination of the cavity also provides the opportunity to determine any presence of intrauterine neoplasm that may have gone previously undetected, especially if a blind screening technique had been used. The HTA® system provides an initial 2-minute diagnostic hysteroscopy cycle, which can be extended if desired or terminated as soon as the examination is completed. While room temperature saline is circulating, the junction of the sheath with the external cervical os should be visualized to confirm a good seal. It is often helpful to apply a second tenaculum at the 3 or 9 o'clock position to compress the cervix around the sheath. If a patient with a patulous cervix is encountered, a multi-tooth tenaculum as devised for hysteroscopy by Gimpelson can be applied (Figure 12). In the extreme situation, since only room temperature saline has been used thus far, the flow of saline can be inter-

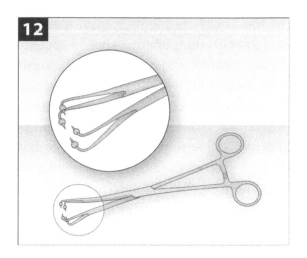

rupted and the sheath temporarily removed to apply an Endo-Loop around the cervix. The HTA® sheath is reinserted and the loop of suture is tightened, providing a purse-string like effect for a very reliable seal around the sheath. Once the examination of the cavity has been completed, the tip of the sheath should be positioned in the lower uterine segment just inside the internal os, where it will remain for the duration of the procedure. Proper position can be confirmed by slowly withdrawing the sheath into the cervical canal until the internal cervical os is visualized. Then the tip of the sheath should be advanced only a few millimeters into the lower uterine segment (Figure 13).

The vaginal speculum should remain in place throughout the procedure to provide easy visualization of the cervix at all times. This will also help avoid contact of the vaginal walls with the sheath. The insulation built into the wall of the sheath prevents it from reaching a harmful temperature, but a patient being treated under minimal anesthesia may sense its warmth and be alarmed. If the flushing cycle has been extended, it must be confirmed that a minimum of 1.5 L of saline remains in the source bag before proceeding with the ablation treatment. This fluid is necessary for cooling the patient and the equipment following the completion of the ablation.

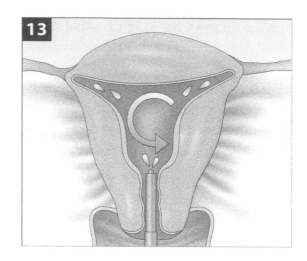

After the flushing and filling cycles have been completed, the message display offers the user the choice to proceed with the treatment. When the "Start" button is pressed to confirm the desire to proceed, the HTA® restarts fluid circulation and gradually increases the temperature of the fluid, requiring approximately three minutes. The volume of fluid in closed-loop circulation is monitored during this period providing the opportunity to detect any defect in the uterine wall, with the detection of a loss of 10 cc of liquid causing fluid circulation to stop and triggering an alarm and message prompt.

During this period, the patient should be monitored for any signs of discomfort and the uterine cavity is continuously visualized to assure that the tip of the sheath remains in the proper position. Once the ablation temperature is reached (message display will indicate between 80–90° C), the system automatically pauses while the system drains a small amount of fluid, and re-establish-

es the fluid level at the '80' mark in the reservoir. The HTA® unit then begins timing the ablation therapy cycle. The message display will show the time required for heating, the duration of ablation, and the time remaining.

Throughout the HTA® therapy cycle, the surgeon watches the hysteroscopic image on the monitor to assure that proper sheath position is maintained. Also, the surgeon should visualize the cervix to confirm that a good seal exists. The temptation and curiosity to look around the cavity or to 'aim' the flow of the saline must be resisted. The surgeon must have faith in the device's ability to properly circulate the heated fluid throughout the cavity due to its nearly 300 cc/minute fluid exchange rate. Manipulation of the sheath during the treatment cycle only increases the chance that a cervical leak may develop, and does nothing to contribute to the effectiveness of the treatment. Occasionally, a bubble may form in part of the uterine cavity, creating an area not in contact with the circulating heated saline. Since a bubble of any appreciable size may insulate tissue from treatment, it should be removed. A simple technique is quite effective; by momentarily pinching the inflow tube (yellow connectors at the pump cassette) the outflow pump action will collapse the uterine cavity within seconds and remove the bubble. When the inflow tube is re-opened, the uterine cavity will refill and the bubble will be gone (Figure 14).

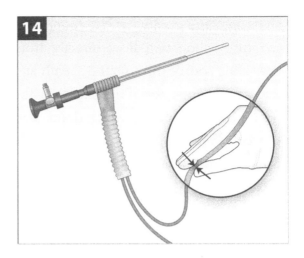

The volume of fluid being circulated in a closed-loop is continuously monitored during fluid warming and the 10-minute therapy cycle to detect any loss of 10 cc of liquid. In the unlikely event that such a loss is detected, the HTA® will immediately interrupt the circulation of the heated fluid. The display of the HTA® will indicate that a 10 cc loss has been detected and will also indicate the rate at which the fluid was lost. This is a key safety feature, since there is a significant difference in risk between a loss at a rate of 2–5 cc/minute compared to a loss at a rate of 100 cc/minute. The indication of a very slow loss can be due to the cavity slowly expanding during simple uterine muscle relaxation. On the other hand, the cause of a sudden loss must be determined before the procedure can be safely continued. If the cause of such a fluid loss cannot be confirmed, the procedure cannot be continued without

significant risk. It is better to proceed directly to the cooling phase and provide additional treatment at a later date, rather than risk serious injury. In any case, the HTA® sheath must never be removed from the patient until after the unit's display indicates that the cooling has been completed and the sheath may be removed from the patient. If the cause of a fluid loss is determined and the decision to safely proceed is made, the therapy cycle can be resumed by pressing "Start." The timer will resume where it left off and continue until completion of the ablation cycle.

Upon completion of the timed ablation cycle, the system will automatically pause and then proceed to the patient cooling cycle. The color of the endometrial lining will change as the procedure progresses (Figure 15). If the procedure is interrupted and terminated by the user, the system will also shift to the patient cooling cycle. When the system shifts into the cooling cycle, room temperature saline will flow directly from the saline source through the sheath and into the uterus; this fluid replaces the hot fluid in the uterus, which drains into the collection bag. This cooling cycle lasts for one minute. When the patient cooling cycle is complete, the digital display will present a message that it is safe to remove the sheath from the patient's uterus and cervix. It is very important that the sheath never be removed from the patient unless this message appears on the message display, or hot fluid may escape into the vagina.

SYSTEM COOLING

After the sheath has been removed from the patient, the HTA® must remain connected to electrical power so that the components can cool. The HTA® continues to flush the hot fluid from the Heater Canister into the drain collection bag.

This process for cooling the external components (heater canister, cassette, reservoir and tubing) continues for several minutes until the temperature in the Heater Canister falls below 45° C. The components of the system should not be handled until the message display indicates that doing so is permitted.

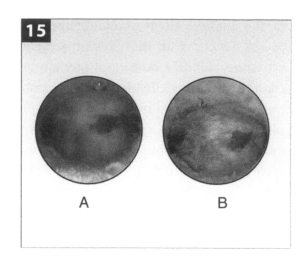

HTA TREATMENT RESULTS

• FDA PHASE III TRIAL
  36 MONTHS POST-TREATMENT
  AMENORRHEA RATE: 53%
  SATISFACTION RATE: 98%

HTA® POST TREATMENT PATIENT MANAGEMENT

Patients may experience a range of postoperative cramping following treatment with the HTA®. In the outpatient surgery setting, pain in the recovery room is usually managed in cooperation with the anesthesia department with the appropriate pain management protocols. Cramps may range from none to significant, but usually last no more than 4–6 hours. All patients to date have reported little or no cramping by 24 hours. Postoperative cramps can usually be relieved with non-steroidal anti-inflammatory drugs (NSAIDS) and it is important for them to be taken according to schedule rather than waiting for pain onset. Our practice is to use ibuprofen 800 mg TID or diclofenac 50 mg TID. We have occasionally used acetaminophen with codeine, Percocet (Endo Pharmaceuticals, Inc., Chadds Ford, PA) or Vicodin (Knoll Pharmaceutical Co., Mount Olive, NJ) postoperatively but rarely after the first 24–48 hours.

For several weeks after the HTA® procedure, the patient may experience a vaginal discharge as typical with all forms of endometrial ablation, which may vary from clear to serosanguineous to brown. She may also experience some menstrual-like bleeding. The bleeding is usually not heavier than a normal period. A postoperative visit can be scheduled in two weeks, at which time, if there is suspicion of hematometra due to cervical stenosis, an endovaginal ultrasound can be performed or the cervix can be sounded and dilated. An argument could be made for routine sounding or dilation at the first postoperative visit for this purpose.

Patients should be reminded that endometrial ablation is not a sterilization procedure and subsequent pregnancy is possible. All patients who are not surgically sterile or who do not have surgically sterile partners should be instructed to use a form of birth control. If a pregnancy should occur, certain risks such as ectopic pregnancy and miscarriage are increased.

Infection following the HTA® procedure is rare, but patients should be instructed to call the office if they experience a temperature greater than 100.4° F. All patients with an elevated temperature or lower abdominal pain should be promptly evaluated in the office.

Following HTA® treatment, some patients will not experience any bleeding at all. Others may experience an endometrial sloughing in months 3 to 6. This may result in heavy bleeding. The patient should be reassured and it should be explained that the bleeding will probably decrease over the following months.

Patients should be instructed to call the office if they experience any of the following symptoms:

increasing abdominal pain, nausea, vomiting or diarrhea, fever, abdominal swelling, cyclic pelvic pain without bleeding and/or bleeding heavier than a normal period.

Any of these symptoms should prompt a thorough evaluation of the patient in a timely fashion.

At 36 months posttreatment, patients treated with the HTA® during its FDA Phase III multi-center trial, reported an amenorrhea rate of 53% and a satisfaction rate of 98%. There has been considerable clinical experience since the FDA approval for marketing of the HTA® system in the United States, with over 16,000 patients treated through mid-2003. This confirms the long-term durability of the outcome of this treatment.

SUGGESTED READING:

Corson SL. A multicenter evaluation of endometrial ablation by Hydro ThermAblator and rollerball for treatment of menorrhagia. J Am Assoc Gynecol Laparosc 2001;8:359-367

Glasser MH, Zimmerman JD. The Hydro ThermAblator system for management of menorrhagia in women with submucous myomas: 12- to 20-month follow-up. J Am Assoc Gynecol Laparosc 2003;10(4):521-527

Goldrath MH, Barrionuevo M, Hussain M. Endometrial ablation by hysteroscopic installation of hot saline solution. J Am Assoc Gynecol Laparosc 1997;4:234-240

Goldrath MH. Evaluation of Hydro ThermAblator and rollerball endometrial ablation for menorrhagia 3 years after treatment. J Am Assoc Gynecol Laparosc 2003;10(4):505-511

Loffer FD. Three-year comparison of thermal balloon and rollerball ablation in treatment of menorrhagia. J Am Assoc Gynecol Laparosc 2001;8:48-54

Richart RM, Botacini das Dores G, Nicolau SM, et al. Histologic studies of the effects of circulating hot saline on the uterus before hysterectomy. J Am Assoc Gynecol Laparosc 1999;6:269-273

MICROWAVE ENDOMETRIAL ABLATION

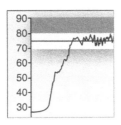

Kevin G. Cooper, M.Sc, M.D., M.R.C.O.G.

Microwave endometrial ablation (MEA™) is a second generation, blind endometrial ablative technique developed and pioneered in the UK in the mid 1990's. It causes no bleeding and does not require fluid distension of the uterine cavity, negating two of the problems associated with first generation hysteroscopic methods. To date, more than 15,000 treatments have been performed worldwide, principally in the UK, Canada, and Australia. The microwave endometrial ablation (or MEA™ system), having completed the necessary evaluation, received U.S. FDA approval in September 2003.

MICROWAVE ENERGY

Microwave ablation should not to be confused with radio frequency endometrial ablation (RaFEA), which was misnamed "microwave" by some sources. Microwaves are electromagnetic waves with a wavelength of 0.3 cm to 30 cm and frequency, 300 to 300,000 Mhz (between radiowaves and infrared radiation) (Figure 1). At a frequency of 9.2 GHz, and at a low power of 30 W, microwave energy predictably and effectively ensures the 5–6 mm depth of necrosis, which is required to completely destroy the basal layer of the endometrium. A microwave generator, or magnetron, supplies microwave energy to a hand held applicator (Figure 2). The applicator is an 8 mm diameter, 15 cm circular metal tube with a dielectric filled waveguide to propagate microwave energy at 9.2 GHz into the uterine cavity (Figure 3). The dielectric waveguide extends beyond the end of the tube to form the radiating tip. With power levels of 30 W, energies of 1.5–9.3 kJ result, and a hemispherical field pattern emanates from the dielectric tip, which if placed in egg white, causes a symmetrical ball of coagulum of constant thickness (Figure 4). Extensive pre-clinical testing undertaken on animal tissue, excised perfused uteri and pre-hysterectomy in vivo spec-

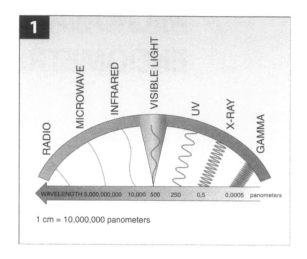

1 cm = 10,000,000 panometers

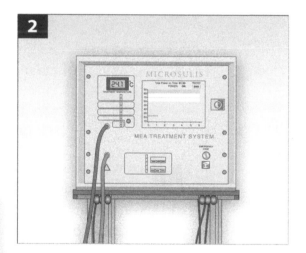

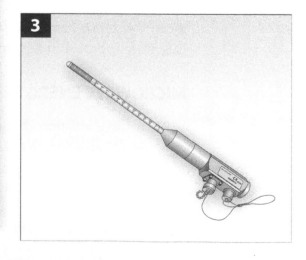

MICROWAVE ENDOMETRIAL ABLATION

- INDICATIONS: TREATMENT OF DUB IN UTERI 6–14 CM, UTERINE WALL THICKNESS MUST BE > 8MM, IRREGULAR CAVITIES OK, FIBROIDS <5CM OK
- PREOP THINNING: OCPs & DANOCRINE – OK, GNRH AGONIST – ?, CURETTAGE – NO
- ANESTHESIA: GENERAL, REGIONAL, LOCAL
- EQUIPMENT: MICROWAVE GENERATOR & MEA DISPOSABLE KIT, GAS HYSTEROSCOPY, DILATORS
- AVERAGE TREATMENT TIME: 3.5 MIN

imens determined that a depth of necrosis of 5–6 mm is consistently achieved.

Uterine tissue has a very high water content so the microwave field amplitude is reduced by about 90% approximately 3 mm from the surface of the applicator tip. Beyond this zone of intense microwave heating, further tissue destruction occurs by thermal conduction from the heated region (Figure 5). The total depth of necrosis depends upon the power level used and the length of time it is applied. The pattern of heating at the tip is hemispherical and monitoring the temperature of the adjacent tissue allows control over the depth of necrosis. A sensor the applicator tip measures the temperature at the surface of the endometrium. A second temperature sensor is (or thermocouple) located at the base of the applicator serves as a control to show a temperature gradient. The temperature at the tip is displayed graphically allowing the surgeon to monitor the process of heating and hence treatment. The system computer screen provides the surgeon with a proven temperature band of 70-80° C (Figure 6). An alarm is activated if the temperature exceeds 85° C and automatically shuts off power at 90° C. Another safety feature is that potential perforation can be determined quickly by a failure to establish a temperature gradient if an attempt to activate the machine is made, resulting in a safety cut out. No grounding is required and there is no dissemination of energy at

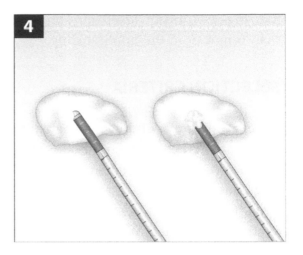

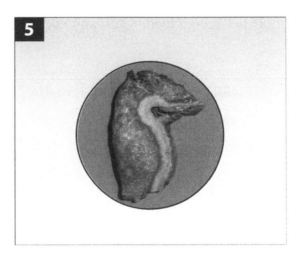

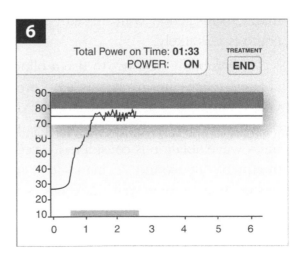

the pre-set power levels any further than 6 mm from the applicator tip.

SELECTION CRITERIA

As with any endometrial ablative technique certain criteria must be satisfied before the procedure is performed. The patient should have excessive menstrual loss for which she desires a surgical treatment; failed medical treatment is not a necessity. Potential patients should be aware that amenorrhea cannot be guaranteed with any ablative

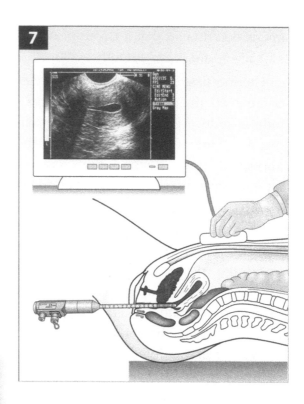

GENERIC SELECTION CRITERIA:

• FAMILY IS COMPLETE;

• ENDOMETRIAL ATYPIA IS EXCLUDED;

• NO ACTIVE GENITAL TRACT INFECTION.

technique and that lighter periods are the likely outcome. If this is understood then dissatisfaction with menstrual outcome is less likely.

It is probably best not to use a blind ablative technique in patients with previous surgery, e.g. myomectomy, or damage to the body of the uterus. If microwave ablation is considered, a pretreatment ultrasound is mandatory to ensure that uterine wall thickness is a minimum of 8 mm (Figure 7). This is most easily done at initial investigation when obtaining the necessary endome-

trial biopsy. If the uterine wall thickness is less than 8 mm then blind ablative techniques are probably inadvisable, particularly without concurrent laparoscopic control. Hysteroscopy is not necessary as an initial investigation (it will be performed immediately prior to insertion of the MEA™ probe) unless to determine whether access to the cavity beyond a submucous fibroid is possible.

ENDOMETRIAL PREPARATION

Endometrial preparation can be undertaken preoperatively with GnRH analogues, but cervical resistance is significantly increased which can be problematic if plans are to undertake the procedure under local anesthesia. It is possible that menstrual outcomes are improved for endometrial ablations following GnRH preparation, although this has not been demonstrated for MEA™. Since microwave ablation requires no fluid-distending medium and bleeding does not occur, the need for excessive thinning is reduced. In vivo studies have clearly shown that the consistent depth of endomyometrial destruction of MEA™ is not compromised at on endometrial thickness less than 10 mm. Microwave ablation should preferably be done when there is no active bleeding as there is a theoretical risk of reduced efficacy. One advantage of endometrial preparation is that the operation can be scheduled accurately when there is no bleeding and with endometrial thickness of less than 10 mm. This can be easily achieved using four to six weeks of Danocrine 400 mg a day, or even the combined oral contraceptive pill. An alternative is to undertake the procedure between day 5 and 10 of the menstrual cycle proliferative phase. Endometrial thickness up to day 10 of the proliferative phase is consistently < 10 mm. This is a convenient technique if a weekly treatment clinic with open access is available. If not, then progestogens can be used to initiate a withdrawal bleed at the desired time so that treatment is scheduled between day 5 and 10 of the withdrawal bleed. An example would be to schedule for two weeks after a five-day course of progestogens.

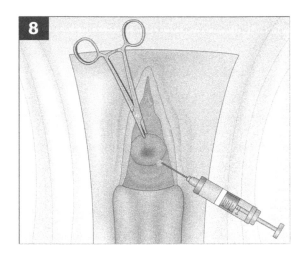

Mechanical preparation of the endometrium is contraindicated either by curettage or suction as there is a risk of wall damage and perforation. This may not be detected prior to treatment with the MEA™ resulting in potential extrauterine thermal damage. Also bleeding and transudate caused by mechanical preparation may reduce the effectiveness of the microwave treatment.

TECHNIQUE

The procedure can be performed under general or local anesthesia. As postoperative pain is accentuated by prostaglandin release, 50 mg of diclofenac may be taken, if not contraindicated. Intravenous access is always recommended and if local anesthesia is to be used a small dose of midazolam (2–4 mg) can be used as an anxiolytic. The cervix is infiltrated using a four quadrant intracervical block at points 2, 4, 8 and 10 o'clock

MEA™ SPECIFIC CRITERIA:

- Uterine wall thickness > 8 mm;
- Cavity length ≤12 cm;
- Irregular cavities can be treated;
- Non-obstructing fibroids < 5cm can be treated;
- Not recommended for repeat procedures.

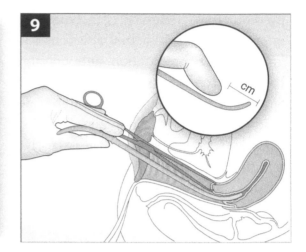

(Figure 8), using a short to medium term acting local anesthetic agent with adrenaline. Over 95% of cases will be completed successfully without recourse to general anesthetic by using this technique.

The cervix is then dilated to 9 mm and the length of the cavity measured (Figure 9). Hysteroscopy is undertaken to identify the endometrial cavity and exclude false passage formation or perforation (Figure 10). This is an essential safety precaution, which should be adopted before undertaking any blind ablative technique. Ultrasound guidance at this point does not exclude false passage formation and is not recommended. The probe, which has centimeter markings on the shaft, is inserted until the tip reaches the fundus, ensuring that the length inserted is the same as that previously measured. The microwave generator is then activated by depressing the foot switch. Once the temperature reaches 70–80° C the probe is moved laterally into the cornual region (Figure 11). The operator aims to main-

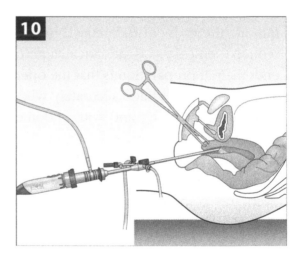

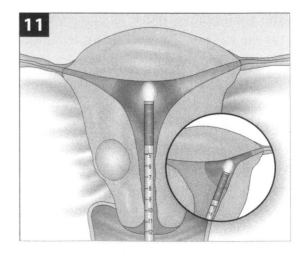

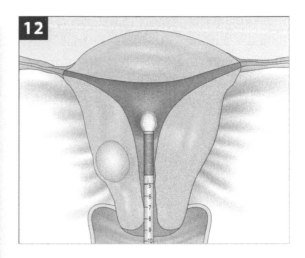

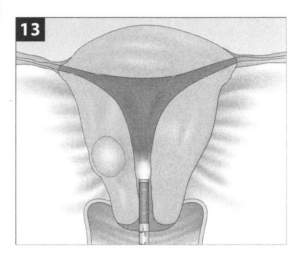

tain the temperature in the white treatment band on the computer screen. The temperature reading will transiently fall, then once the operating temperature is attained again the probe is moved to the opposite cornua and the process repeated. The probe is then gradually withdrawn while maintaining the temperature in the 70–80° C range (Figure 12). This technique effectively "paints" the uterine cavity with a ball of destructive microwave energy to a predictable depth. The treatment phase should be stopped after the yellow colored area stops on the probe shaft (Figure 13).This is set 4 cm from the tip and ensures that the endocervical canal is not treated which could result in stenosis with subsequent hematometra or pain. For women with a shortened cervix due to previous surgery, treatment below the yellow mark can be safely undertaken. The treatment time varies with cavity length, but is usually between 2–4 minutes. Treatment times are also longer if endometrial thickness is increased due to energy absorption and heat sink effect.

WHAT TO EXPECT

Initial results were very encouraging, showing active treatment times of less than three minutes and patient satisfaction rates of above 90%. Short and medium term results have been published. Further randomized trials have demonstrated its acceptability for use under local anesthetic and also the ability to treat in the office setting rather

---

MEA™ RESULTS

- FDA TRIALS
  ONE YEAR POST TREATMENT
  61% AMENORRHEA RATE
  >90% SATISFACTION RATE

- OTHER TRIALS
  40 TO 60% AMENORRHEA RATE

---

than operating room without the need for endometrial preparation. Another multicenter randomized trial has been completed comparing microwave with rollerball ablation in accordance with FDA requirements.

Amenorrhea rates from the randomized trials evaluating MEA™ vary between 40% and 60%, while bleeding and dysmenorrhea scores are markedly improved. Satisfaction and acceptability in treatment levels of over 90% were achieved. Importantly, measurements of health-related quality of life, which are significantly affected by excessive menstrual loss, are returned to normative levels.

The technique is simple to learn; over 90% of treatments in the UK trials were performed by junior (resident) gynecologists, recently trained in the technique. It is undoubtedly quick to perform and is very safe as long as one adheres to the simple guidelines outlined here. Prospective collection of data is ongoing from the independent randomized trials of any complications arising from any users. This should be the objective of any new surgical technique to ensure that its practice is safe and evidence based.

SUGGESTED READING:

Cooper K G, Bain C, Parkin D E. Comparison of microwave endometrial ablation and transcervical resection of the endometrium for treatment of heavy menstrual loss: a randomized trial. Lancet, November 1999;354:1859-63

Hodgson DA, Feldberg IB, Sharp N, Cronin N, Evans M, Hircowitz L. Microwave endometrial ablation: development, clinical trials and outcomes at three years. Br J Obstet Gynaecol 1999;106:684-694

Bain C, Cooper KG, Parkin DE. Microwave endometrial ablation versus endometrial resection: a randomized controlled trial. Obstet Gynecol, 2002;99(6):983-7

Bain C, Cooper K, Parkin D. A partially randomized patient preference trial of microwave endometrial ablation using local anesthesia and intravenous sedation or general anesthesia. Gynecol Endos 2001;10(4):223-228

Parkin D. Microwave endometrial ablation (MEA™): A safe technique? Complication data from a prospective series of 1400 cases. Gynecol Endos 2000;9(6):385-388

Wallage S, Cooper KG, Miller ID. Microwave endometrial ablation: Does endometrial thickness or the medium for pre-operative hysteroscopy affect the depth of ablation? Gynac Endoscopy 2002; 11(2-30): 107-110

ENDOMETRIAL CRYOABLATION

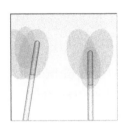

Errico Zupi, M.D.
Alessio Piredda, M.D.
Daniela Marconi, M.D., Ph.D.

C ryoablation of the endometrium is a second generation endometrial ablation technique. Recently Cryogen™, Inc. (San Diego, CA, USA) developed a new effective device called Her Option™ System.

First generation techniques include:

Transcervical resection of the endometrium;

Rollerball ablation;

Endometrial laser ablation.

These techniques required surgical expertise and experience, were potentially dangerous because of use and absorption of distension media, required general anesthesia and had a high number of recurrences because of the difficulty to obtain a complete resection of the endometrium considering the depth of tissue destruction.

Compared to the first generation ablation techniques, second generation have common features. In fact second generation techniques were developed mostly to reduce the level of operator skill without compromising effectiveness. These methods are easy to learn and don't require extensive training.

There are systems related to heat, including water balloon, heated saline, lasers, microwaves, bipolar electrosurgery and systems based on freezing like cryoablation.

ENDOMETRIAL CRYOABLATION

- INDICATIONS: TREATMENT OF DUB, NO LIMITS ON UTERINE SIZE, IRREGULAR CAVITY – OK, SMALL FIBROIDS – OK
- PREOP THINNING: NOT ADVOCATED, BUT NOT CONTRAINDICATED
- ANESTHESIA: GENERAL, REGIONAL, LOCAL
- EQUIPMENT: HER OPTION™ CONSOLE WITH CRYOPROBE, DISPOSABLE PROBE, CATHETER, SALINE, ULTRASOUND
- AVERAGE TREATMENT TIME: 15 MIN

HER OPTION™ CRYOABLATION THERAPY SYSTEM

The Her Option™ Cryoablation Therapy System (Figure 1) is a cryoablation device with a gas cooled Cryoprobe. Its operation is based on the Joule-Thomson principle in which pressurized gas is expanded through a small orifice to produce cooling. The coolant or gas used in the system is a proprietary blend of commonly used coolants, which are non-toxic, non-corrosive, non-flammable and non-CFC.

The system is intended to destroy tissue during ablation procedures by the application of extreme cold at the distal

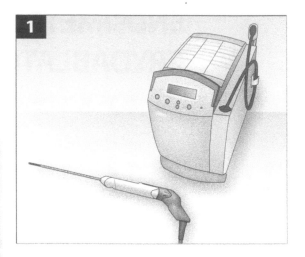

tip of the Cryoprobe. A -20°C temperature is lethal to tissue. The ice front advances through the uterine tissue, creating a CryoZone, rather than expanding within the endometrial cavity.

The System includes a Console, a Cryoprobe and a Disposable Probe. The Cryoprobe with Disposable Probe attached is referred to as the Probe. A compressor housed in the Console is fully charged with coolant and is semi-hermetically sealed prior to shipping to ensure zero leakage. Activation of the System freeze cycle causes gas to exit the compressor and flow to the Probe where it expands to a low pressure across a small diameter orifice at the tip of the Probe. As a result, a rapid temperature drop occurs. This temperature drop is transferred to the tissue-contacting tip of the Disposable Probe, causing freezing. Gas then returns to the compressor and is recirculated. Deactivation of the freeze cycle stops gas flow to the Probe, ending cooling.

CONSOLE

The Console (Figure 2) contains the compressor system that, during operation, continuously circulates a pressurized gas mixture consisting of common refrigerants during operation. The compressor system has an operating pressure of 350 to 400 psi. A pressure control feedback loop controls the stroke of the compressor and limits the pressure to less than 400 psi.

The controls and displays are mounted on the front panel of the Console. There is an on/off button as well as other information for commands and user interface. The user interface will display the cycle, temperature, mode (heating or thawing) and total time in each mode.

CRYOPROBE

The Cryoprobe consists of a handle and a probe shaft. Flexible plastic transport hoses connect the Cryoprobe to the compressor system housed within the Console. The Cryoprobe shaft is comprised of concentrically oriented stainless steel tubes and a metal tip. Two of the stainless steel tubes form the walls of the device. The device provides insulation to prevent freezing along its length by evacuation of the space between the outer and middle tubes to a pressure less than 1 microtorr. The remaining tubes deliver the high-pressure gas to the metal tip. Pressurized inflow gas is carried through the lumen

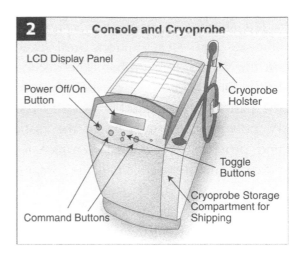

Console and Cryoprobe

- LCD Display Panel
- Power Off/On Button
- Cryoprobe Holster
- Toggle Buttons
- Cryoprobe Storage Compartment for Shipping
- Command Buttons

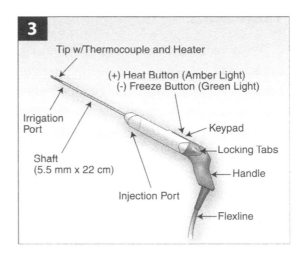

- Tip w/Thermocouple and Heater
- (+) Heat Button (Amber Light)
- (-) Freeze Button (Green Light)
- Irrigation Port
- Keypad
- Shaft (5.5 mm x 22 cm)
- Locking Tabs
- Handle
- Injection Port
- Flexline

of the innermost tube and the expanded effluent gas is returned through the annular space between the inner and middle tubes. The tip at the distal end of the shaft is the site of the freezing (Figure 3).

DISPOSABLE PROBE (ALSO CALLED THE DISPOSABLE CONTROL UNIT)

The Disposable Probe (Figure 4) fits snugly over the Cryoprobe. It is provided sterile, for single use only. The "Freeze" and "Heat" buttons are located on this Disposable Probe. The portion of the Disposable Probe which contacts the patient is fabricated from USP Class IV polymers. A metal tip at the distal end provides a conductive surface for efficient heat transfer. This tip contains the heater wire and thermocouple. The heater is used at the completion of a freeze cycle to ease removal of the tip from the iceball.

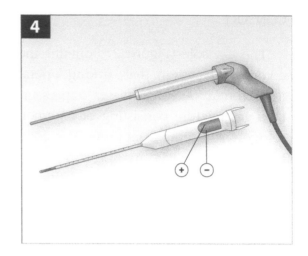

TECHNIQUE

With patients under general or local anesthesia, a Foley catheter is inserted into the bladder and the bladder filled with 300 to 400 mL saline to facilitate ultrasound visualization during the procedure. Filling of the bladder is done prior to insertion of the probe. If necessary, the endocervical canal is dilated to accommodate the 5.5 mm cryosurgical probe. The probe is then inserted and used as a uterine sound to determine maximum length of the fundus. Probe placement to the fundus is confirmed by transabdominal ultrasound (Figures 5, 6).

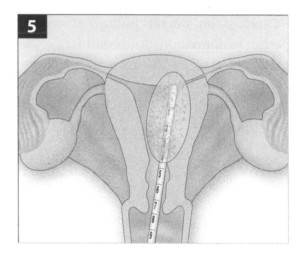

The Probe is then angled toward one cornua. A hollow injection tubing present in the Probe allows fluid to be instilled into the uterine cavity. Sterile saline (5 mL) is injected into the uterine cavity to couple the probe thermally to tissue. Transabdominal ultrasound will allow visualization of fluid instillation. The first freeze begins and continues for

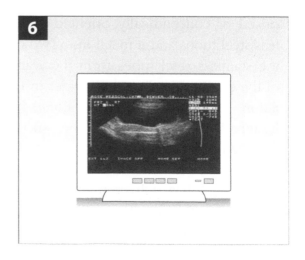

CRYOABLATION TECHNIQUE

- FOLEY: FILL BLADDER WITH 300 CC SALINE
- INSERT PROBE TO FUNDUS & ULTRASOUND
- INSTILL 5 CC SALINE INTO UTERINE CAVITY PRIOR TO EACH FREEZE
- BEGIN 1ST FREEZE (4 MIN) IN CORNUA, MEASURE ICEBALL EVERY 1 MIN
- 2ND FREEZE (6 MIN) IN OPPOSITE CORNUA
- PROBE COOLED TO −90° C, 3.5 TO 5 CM ICEBALL
- 0° C AT EDGE OF ICEBALL, −20° C AT 1.5 CM FROM EDGE
- UTERINE SIZE DETERMINES NUMBER OF ICEBALLS NEEDED

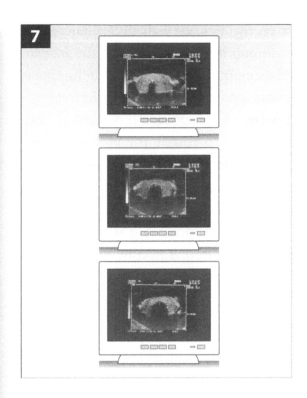

4 minutes. With an abdominal probe (5–7 MHz), an ultrasound technician monitors growth of the ice ball taking transverse measurements of the diameter at 1-minute intervals (Figure 7 – A, B, C). The leading edge of the iceball is easily seen by ultrasound. The distance of the ice front to the serosal surface is measured. After the first freeze is completed the Probe tip is thawed permitting the Probe to disengage from tissue (~1min). A defrost button is pressed on the Probe handle to expedite the thawing process. The Probe is then positioned at the opposite cornua by withdrawing it into the endocervical canal, angling toward the cornua, and reinsert-

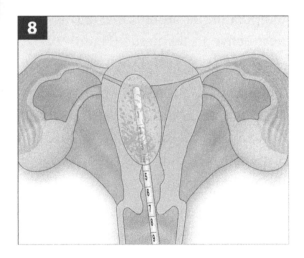

ing it (Figure 8). In some cases it may be necessary to wait for several minutes for the first iceball to melt partially before the Probe can be advanced. In addition, it may be useful to flush with 15 mL of saline before withdrawing the Probe from the first ice ball to facilitate repositioning by helping to melt the iceball. Placement of the Probe on the fundus is confirmed by ultrasound. After repositioning, 5 mL of saline is instilled into the cavity to couple the probe thermally to tissue. The second freeze is begun and continued for 6 minutes. Serial ultrasound is measured as in the first freeze. The increasing size of the iceball can be monitored by ultrasound as seen in Figure 7.

When the probe is cooled to a temperature of less than -90°C, a 3.5–5 cm elliptical iceball forms around the probe.

At the edge of the iceball, the tissue temperature is around 0°C and is nondestructive to the tissue (Figure 9).

A temperature of -20°C, which is lethal to tissue, is reached approximately 1.5 cm from the edge of the iceball, permanently destroying the endometrial tissue, including the basalis layer of the endometrium.

Uterine cavity size determines the number of iceballs necessary to destroy the entire cavity. The entire procedure takes 10 to 20 minutes, depending on the size of the uterine cavity.

Additional Freeze Cycles may be performed (at the midline or at either cornua) at the physician's discretion (Figure 10).

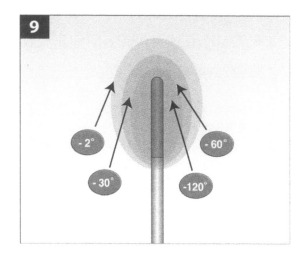

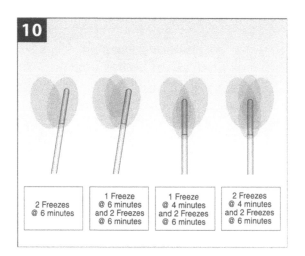

ADVANTAGES OF CRYOABLATION

Cryoablation is not a totally blind procedure. The iceball created can be followed by abdominal ultrasound and the procedure can be stopped when the edge of the iceball approaches the serosa of the uterus. This visual feedback also allows for complete ablation of the entire cavity and is not dependent on the cavity size.

The procedure doesn't need any distension media avoiding any sort of problems due to absorption.

The freezing of tissue causes less pain because of cryoanesthesia. All the other ablation devices utilize heat energy.

The patients experience just minimal uterine cramping during the procedure.

DISADVANTAGES OF CRYOABLATION

Some possible disadvantages could be:

Lack of direct visualization of the uterine cavity;

It should be noted that most ablation techniques based on heat are almost totally blind procedures. Cryoablation procedure as already described may be followed by ultrasound.

Lack of data on the success in patients with intracavitary lesions such as myomata and polyps;

FDA statement: most of the global ablation techniques were tested in patients with normal uterine cavities.

Rutherford in 1998 and Dobak in 2000 utilized endometrial cryoablation even in patients with large intrauterine myomas. They stated that destruction of myomas is equivalent to that of normal myometrium and that the iceball produced by the cryoprobe maintains its circular shape and remains symmetric even in the face of submucosal fibroids.

Potential disadvantage in using endometrial cryoablation to treat submucous fibroids could be the fact that the depth of tissue destruction, ranging from 9 to 15 mm, may lead to an incomplete destruction of myoma tissue and its vascularization. Persistence of a fibroid may lead to a possible relapse of meno/metrorrhagia.

Absence of pathological specimens:

Before treatment patients should be carefully studied.

The Pre-op work up should include: history and complete physical examination, including pelvic exam; negative PAP smear and endometrial biopsy to rule out cervical or endometrial malignancy and pre-malignant changes to the uterus; sonography, hysteroscopy, hysterosalpingography or any other indicated diagnostic tests or procedures that might uncover a possible cause for menorrhagia within six months of performing the procedure.

RESULTS OF THE TECHNIQUE

Townsend et al. recently published the two years follow up results of a randomized multicenter trial in which 272 patients underwent an ablative procedure.

Patients were divided in two groups depending on the kind of treatment: cryoablation group and electroablation group.

At 24 months follow up, 94% of cryoablation and 93% of electroablation patients no longer had abnormal uterine bleeding.

At 24 months, 77% of the cryoablation group reported that menstrual pain was nonexistent or much improved versus 81% of the electroablation group. Premenstrual syndrome symptoms were absent or mild at 24 months in 67% of cryoablation and 79% of electroablation patients. At 24 months, 91% of cryoablation patients were very or extremely satisfied with treatment results compared with 88% of electroablation patients.

Of the cryoablation group, 13 patients (7.0%) proceeded to hysterectomy and 5 (2.7%) to repeat ablation compared with 7 (8.1%) and 1 (1.2%) of the electroablation group, respectively. The median time at risk for retreatment was 20.7 months (range, 0.5–31.3 months). The retreatment rate at 30 months was similar for the cryoablation (12.9%) and electroablation (14.0%) groups (Figure 11).

Both cryoablation and electroablation were associated with a high success in

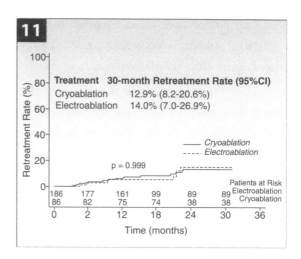

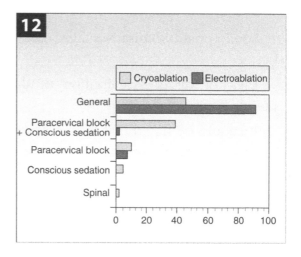

CRYOABLATION RESULTS

- ONE 2YR MULTICENTER RANDOMIZED TRIAL (TOWNSEND, ET AL)
  91% SATISFACTION RATE
  94% REPORTED DECREASED BLEEDING
  77% REPORTED DECREASED PAIN

treatment of DUB. Both led to improvements in pain, self-perceived symptoms of PMS, mood, and quality of life. Cryoablation was accomplished with significantly less anesthesia than electroablation (Figure 12).

Several arguments point at cryoablation as potentially preferred over electroablation: technical ease of the procedure, less anesthesia requirement, and avoidance of potential complications related to distention medium during electroablation. Furthermore, ultrasound guidance provides the operator with real-time, three-dimensional assessment of the uterus and depth of tissue freezing in relation to anatomic landmarks such as uterine serosa. Ultrasonographic guidance is an important safety feature as it facilitates observation of the leading edge of the ice front. Comparable monitoring of depth of tissue destruction is not available in procedures relying on heating, such as electroablation, heated fluids, lasers, or microwaves.

The leading edge of the ice front is at temperatures in the range of $-1°$ to $-2°$ C and is not destructive. Necrosis occurs at $-15°$ to $-20°$ C. Studies on extirpated uteri as well as prehysterectomy cryoablations showed that tissue necrosis lags approximately 3 to 4 mm behind the ice front. These characteristics of tissue response to freezing further enhance the safety of Cryoablation. The ability to monitor the extent of tissue ablation in real time allows freezing protocols to be developed according to an individual patient's uterine architecture. Thus, in contrast to some global ablation devices, cryoablation can be accomplished in irregularly shaped uteri.

Another important benefit of Cryoablation with Her Option™ system is the greatly reduced need for anesthesia. At least two factors contribute to minimal intraoperative discomfort: dilatation of the cervix is rarely required, and tissue freezing, in contrast to heating, has analgesic properties. The experiences of several centers participating in this study demonstrate that the Her Option™ system is ideally suited to performing endometrial ablation in the office setting under paracervical block.

Endometrial cryoablation with Her Option™ System is a flexible, safe, and reliable treatment of DUB. The analgesic properties of tissue freezing in combination with a small-diameter cryoprobe minimize intraoperative discomfort.

SUGGESTED READING:

Cahan W. Cryosurgery of the uterine cavity. Am J Obstet Gynecol 1967;99:138–53

Sowter M C. New surgical treatments for menorrhagia. Lancet 2003;361:1456–58

Dobak J D., Willems J., Howard R., Shea C., Townsend D. E. Endometrial Cryoablation with Ultrasound Visualization in Women Undergoing Hysterectomy. J Am Assoc Gynecol Laparosc 2000;7:(1):89–93

Rutherford T J, Zreik T G, Troiano R N, et al: Endometrial Cryoablation, A Minimally Invasive Procedure For Abnormal Uterine Bleeding. J Am Assoc Gynecol Laparosc 1998;5(1):23–28

Townsend D E, Duleba A J, Wilke M. Durability of treatment effects after endometrial cryoablation versus rollerball electroablation for normal uterine bleeding: two-year results of a multicenter randomized trial. Am J Obstet Gynecol 2003;188:699-701

Smith J J, Fraser J An estimation of tissue damage and thermal history in the cryolesion. Cryobiology 1974;11:139-147

Doak JD, Willems J. Extirpated uterine endometrial cryoablation with ultrasound visualization. J Am Assoc Gynecol Laparosc 2000;7:(1):95–101

Evans P J. Cryoanalgesia. The application of low temperatures to nerves to produce anaesthesia or analgesia. Anestesia 1981;36:1003-1013

Duleba J A, Martha C H, Soderstrom R M, Townsend D.E. A randomized study comparing endometrial cryoablation and rollerball electroablation for treatment of dysfunctional uterine bleeding. J Am Assoc Gynecol Laparosc 2003;10(1):17–26

NOVASURE™ GLOBAL ENDOMETRIAL ABLATION

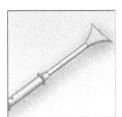

Jay M. Cooper, M.D.
Eugene V. Skalnyi, M.D.

Radio Frequency (RF) energy has been successfully employed with the use of "First Generation" (i.e., hysteroscopic) endometrial ablation systems (rollerball, loop, and rollerbar). With the development of "Second Generation" products, this time tested energy found an application as well.

NOVASURE™ TECHNOLOGY OVERVIEW

The NovaSure™ System consists of a disposable ablation device, portable RF controller, desiccant, foot switch, and power cord (Figure 1). The disposable device consists of a single-patient use, conformable bipolar electrode array mounted on an expandable frame (Figure 2). The 7.2 mm diameter device is inserted trans-cervically into the uterine cavity. The protective sheath is then retracted to allow the bipolar electrode array to be deployed and conform to the uterine cavity. The electrode array consists of a gold-plated, porous fabric mesh through which steam and moisture are continuously suctioned as tissue is desiccated.

NOVASURE™

- INDICATION: TREATMENT OF DUB IN UTERI <10 CM
- PREOP THINNING: NO PRETREATMENT NEEDED
- ANESTHESIA: GENERAL, REGIONAL, LOCAL
- EQUIPMENT: NOVASURE™ RF CONTROLLER & DISPOSABLE DEVICE, SPECULUM, TENACULUM, UTERINE SOUND, DILATORS
- AVERAGE TREATMENT TIME: 90 SEC

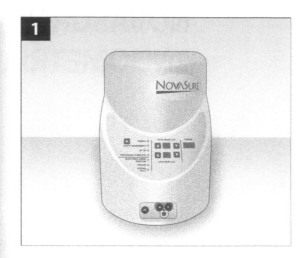

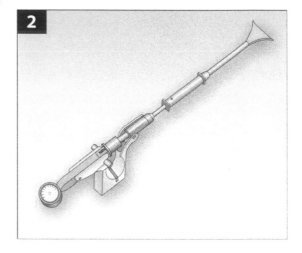

The disposable device works in conjunction with a dedicated RF Controller to perform a customized, global endometrial ablation in an average treatment time of 90 seconds. There is no need for concomitant hysteroscopic visualization or endometrial pre-treatment of any kind. The specific configuration of the electrode array and the predetermined power (specific to the patient's uterine cavity size) delivered by the Controller create a confluent tapered depth of ablation characterized by a deeper ablation in the main body of the uterus and a more shallow ablation profile in the regions of the cornua and internal cervical os (Figure 3). The Controller automatically calculates the required power output based on the patient's uterine cavity length and width. Intra-operative uterine sounding measurements allow assessment of the length of the cavity, whereas the

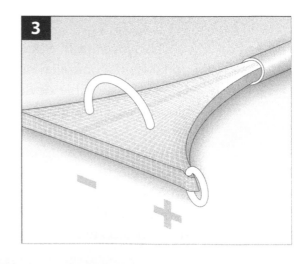

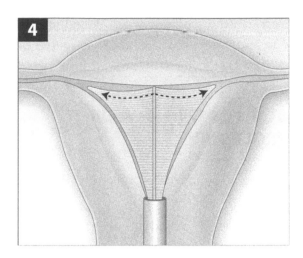

NovaSure™ disposable device measures the uterine cavity width (cornu-to-cornu distance) (Figure 4). The operator key enters these measurements into the RF Controller. A patented Moisture Transport Vacuum System contained within the Controller creates and maintains vacuum in the uterine cavity throughout the ablation procedure, assuring constant apposition between the electrode array and the endometrium, while simultaneously allowing for the continuous removal of ablation bi-products during the treatment.

The Cavity Integrity Assessment System is an integral part of the NovaSure™ System. This automatic safety feature was developed and implemented to assist the physician in the timely detection of uterine wall perforation, such as might be caused by sounding and/or dilation, thus preventing energy delivery. Utilizing a hysteroflator-type technology, CO_2 from a cartridge on the back of the controller is delivered into the uterine cavity at a safe flow rate and pressure. When an intrauterine CO_2 pressure of 50 mmHg is reached and maintained for 4 seconds, thereby confirming good uterine wall integrity, the controller allows the ablation process to proceed.

During the ablation, the flow of RF energy vaporizes the endometrium regardless of its thickness. As the ablation process continues, the underlying superficial myometrium is also desiccated and coagulated. As tissue destruction reaches the optimal depth for a safe and effective ablation, an increase in tissue impedance to 50 ohms causes the Controller to terminate power delivery, thereby providing a self-regulating process. Continuous monitoring of tissue impedance during the ablation process automatically controls the depth of endomyometrial ablation.

NOVASURE SYSTEM SET-UP

Set-up of the NovaSure™ system is very simple and can be easily accomplished by a single individual in 1–2 minutes. The NovaSure™ RF controller is connected to a source of electrical power and turned on using the toggle switch in the back. The CO_2 regulator is then opened to "HI." The pneumatic footswitch is connected to the front panel of the controller. The NovaSure™ disposable device is removed from the sterile package and non-sterile filter desiccant is connected to the proximal portion of the suction line. Plugging the NovaSure™ device into the front panel of the RF controller completes the set-up.

STEPS OF THE NOVASURE™ PROCEDURE

The NovaSure™ procedure is performed as follows:

Following a pelvic examination, a vaginal speculum is inserted. The anterior lip of the cervix is grasped with a tenaculum. The cavity is sounded and the uterine sound measurement is taken (Figure 5). During cervical dilation to 7.5–8 mm, the length of the cervix is assessed by measuring the distance between the internal and external cervical os. In the vast majority of patients, cervical dilation is associated with a resistance encountered during the passage of the distal tip of a Hegar dilator through the internal cervical os (Figure 6). As soon as this resistance is felt, advancement of the dilator should be stopped and a finger should be placed on the dilator at the level of the external cervical os. The Hegar dilator is then withdrawn and the length from its distal tip to the noted location on the shaft of the dilator is measured. The length of the uterine cavity is then calculated (fundus-to-internal os) by subtracting the cervical length from the sounding length. This calculated value represents the length of the uterine cavity that will be subjected to ablation. The same cal-

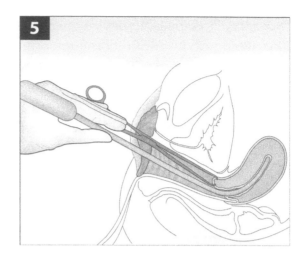

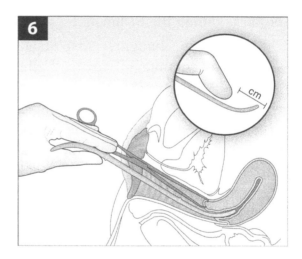

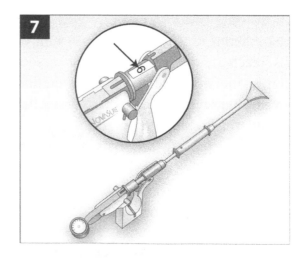

culated value of the uterine cavity length is then set on the disposable NovaSure™ device (Figure 7). This feature will allow for exposure of the electrode to the required length. The NovaSure™ disposable device is then inserted, the handles squeezed and locked to deploy the electrode array, and the instrument is then properly seated in the uterine cavity (Figure 8). The seating procedure must be performed in order for the bi-polar electrode to find its optimal position in the uterine cavity.

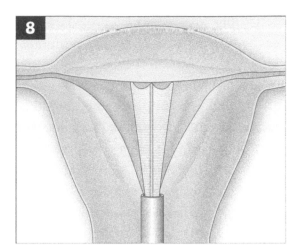

The operator performs the seating procedure using the following motions:

First, the handles of the device are moved up and down to accommodate for antero- or retro- position of the axis of the uterus (Figure 9);

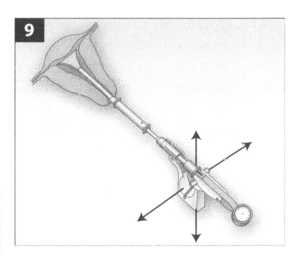

NOVASURE™ TECHNIQUE

- SET-UP IS EASY, REQUIRES < 2 MIN.
- CALCULATE UTERINE CAVITY LENGTH
- ELECTRODE ARRAY IS "SEATED" IN THE UTERINE CAVITY YIELDING UTERINE CAVITY WIDTH
- LENGTH & WIDTH ENTERED IN RF CONTROLLER
- CERVICAL COLLAR APPLIED
- CAVITY INTEGRITY ASSESSMENT TEST
- MOISTURE TRANSPORT VACUUM SYSTEM
- RF ENERGY COAGULATES UP TO 50 OHMS IMPEDANCE

The handles are then moved laterally to the left and to the right to accommodate for any lateral displacement of the cavity axis;

The handles of the device are then gently rotated 45° counterclockwise and 45° clockwise (Figure 10);

The device is then pulled back slightly and then advanced firmly to the fundus to complete the seating procedure.

During the seating procedure, the cavity width reading will continuously increase as indicated by the width dial (Figure 11). As mentioned in the steps above, the seating procedure should be repeated until a maximum value has been reached and no increase in width value is observed with continued attempts to seat the device.

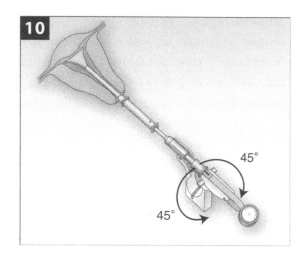

The cavity length value (sound measurement minus length of the cervix) and cavity width value are key-entered into the RF Controller to allow for a precise and automatic calculation of the power output required for an optimal ablation of the cavity of this size. The cervical collar (Figure 12) is then advanced to the cervix and locked in place to create an airtight seal.

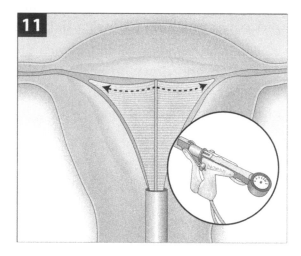

A single tap on the pneumatic footswitch initiates the automatic Cavity Integrity Assessment Test (perforation detection cycle), which lasts on average 8nseconds. The Cavity Integrity Assessment Test is associated with an audible tone and a flashing green "Cavity Assessment" LED light. Upon successful completion of this test, the LED becomes solid green and the audible tone stops. The RF Controller is engaged by pressing the "Enable" button and a second single tap of the footswitch starts the ablation cycle. During the ablation cycle a bright blue "RF On" LED is illuminated (Figure 13). At the end of the ablation cycle the RF Controller automatically terminates energy delivery and a green "Procedure

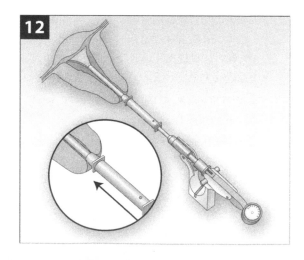

Complete" LED is illuminated. The NovaSure™ device is unlocked, closed, and then device is withdrawn from the uterine cavity. The tenaculum and vaginal speculum are removed to conclude the procedure.

TROUBLESHOOTING

Alarm conditions are very infrequent during the NovaSure™ endometrial ablation procedure, but they may occur. The most common alarm is associated with the Cavity Integrity Assessment Test and inability to pass the perforation detection test due to failure to adequately pressurize the uterine cavity. This alarm is associated with an audible sound and illumination of a solid red "Cavity Assessment" LED. The audible

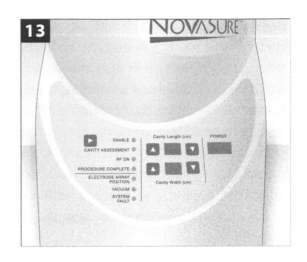

• ASSESSMENT TEST: IN THE VAST MAJORITY OF CASES THIS CAN BE ACCOMPLISHED BY ADVANCING FORWARD THE CERVICAL COLLAR TO THE CERVIX AND LOCKING IT IN PLACE;

THE FOLLOWING TROUBLESHOOTING STEPS SHOULD BE UNDERTAKEN:

• CHECK THE LINES OF THE DEVICE, MAKING SURE THE DEVICE LUER-LOCKS ARE TIGHT, AND TO ASSURE A TIGHT CONNECTION OF THE LINES TO THE DESICCANT;

• THE OPERATOR SHOULD MAKE CERTAIN THAT HIS/HER STOOL IS NOT PLACED ON THE LINE OF THE DEVICE;

• A GOOD SEAL AT THE CERVIX IS REQUIRED IN ORDER TO SUCCESSFULLY PASS THE CAVITY INTEGRITY;

alarm can be stopped by pressing the foot-switch. A second tap of the foot-switch will initiate another perforation detection test.

An inadequate seal of the cervix may result in the appearance of CO_2 bubbles at the cervix and/or hissing sound of gas escaping from the uterine cavity.

If no leakage of gas is observed at the cervix and the lines have been checked, there is a very high probability of a perforation. The integrity of the uterine wall should be assessed with the use of hysteroscopy. The fact that no visible perforation can be identified does not mean that the integrity of the uterine wall has not been breached. The perforation detection system is very sensitive and is capable of identifying a perforation as small as that created with an 18-gauge needle in 100% of cases. If the perforation detection test cannot be passed the system will lock and not allow the operator to proceed with the ablation and the procedure should be aborted.

CLINICAL RESULTS

A significant number of clinical trials have been conducted worldwide in order to assess the safety, efficacy, and other attributes of the NovaSure™ system (Figure 14).

A large multicenter, international randomized clinical trial was conducted in support of the PMA application (FDA trial) and included 265 pre-menopausal women with excessive menstrual bleeding due to benign causes. In this clinical trial, the NovaSure™ system treatment group (175 patients) was compared to a control group of patients treated with loop resection followed by a rollerball ablation (90 patients).

Two-year follow-up results showed that the two treatment modalities were effective in reducing excessive menstrual blood loss. Some 98% of the NovaSure™ patients and 92% of the rollerball patients reported normal bleeding or less pictorial blood loss-

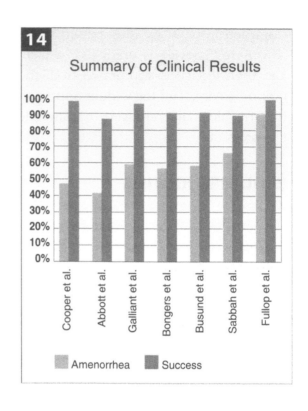

assessment chart ((PBLAC) scores < 100) at 2-year post-treatment. In-patients with 24-month follow-up, 47% of the NovaSure™ patients and 35% of the rollerball patients experienced amenorrhea. Treatment time, defined as the length of time during which RF energy is delivered, averaged 84 seconds in the NovaSure™ Group. Some 73% of the NovaSure™ patients had the procedure performed under local and/or IV sedation, while 82% of the rollerball patients were treated utilizing general or epidural anesthesia. The only adverse event observed in the NovaSure™ arm was a single case of bradycardia. In contrast, 3 uterine perforations and 3 cervical tears were observed in the rollerball arm.

There was a significant decrease in premenstrual symptoms and dysmenorrhea in both treatment groups at 24 months following the procedure. Based on the results obtained in this clinical trial, the FDA determined that the NovaSure™ system was both safe and effective and approved it for sale in the US in 2001.

Additional clinical trials of note include the following:

• Abott, et al. conducted a randomized, double blind clinical trial comparing the NovaSure™ with the Cavaterm system. Amenorrhea and satisfaction rates reported in the NovaSure™ arm at the 12-month follow-up were 43% and 92%, respectively, compared to 11% and 83% in the Cavaterm group, respectively.

• Bongers, et al. conducted a randomized, double blind clinical trial comparing the efficacy of the NovaSure™ system with the ThermaChoice balloon. Amenorrhea and satisfaction rates observed in the NovaSure™ group at the 12-month follow-up were 55% and 94%, respectively, compared to 8% and 77% in the ThermaChoice group.

• Gallinat, et al. reported the results of a 107 patient prospective clinical trial. The amenorrhea rate achieved in women undergoing the NovaSure™ procedure was 58% at 12-month follow-up, with a 96.1% success rate. At 3-years follow-up the reported amenorrhea in this series of patients was 65% with 97% being considered successful.

• Busund, et al. conducted a multi-center, prospective study in which 58% of patients undergoing NovaSure™ ablation reported amenorrhea. A reduction of menstrual bleeding to normal levels at 12-month follow-up was reported in 91.5% of patients.

• Fulop, et al. reported a 90% amenorrhea rate and a 100% success rate in reduction of bleeding to normal levels in 75 patients followed for 3 years.

• Laberge, et al. conducted a clinical trial comparing the intra- and postoperative pain associated with use of the NovaSure™ and ThermaChoice systems. The use of NovaSure™ system was associated with statistically significant lower intra- and postoperative pain level when compared with the use of the ThermaChoice system.

Based upon data generated from this large number of clinical trials, the NovaSure™ system has been demonstrated to be extraordinarily safe and effective, yielding high amenorrhea success and patient satisfaction rates. This endometrial ablation system should be strongly considered as a treatment modality of choice in patients with excessive uterine bleeding to avoid hysterectomy.

SUGGESTED READING:

Laberge P. NovaSure™ Technology Overview. Proceedings of the Second World Congress on Controversies in Obstetrics, Gynecology & Infertility, Vol. I, Paris, France 2001; pp 303-310

Cooper J, Brill A, Fullop T. Is endometrial pre-treatment necessary in NovaSure™ 3-D endometrial ablation. Gynaecol Endosc 2001;10(3):179-182

Gallinat A. Carbon Dioxide Hysteroscopy: Principles and Physiology. In: Hysteroscopy Principles and Practice, AM Siegler, HJ Lindemann, (eds.) Philadelphia, J. B. Lippincott 1984, pp. 45-47

Cooper J. NovaSure™ GEA Technology Overview. Analysis of Worldwide Clinical Results. Proceedings of the Second World Congress on Controversies in Obstetrics, Gynecology & Infertility Vol. I, Paris, France 2001;pp 311-318

Cooper J, Gimpelson R, Laberge P, Galen D, Garza-Leal JG, Scott J, Leyland N, Martyn P, Liu J. A randomized, multicenter trial of safety and efficacy of the NovaSure™ system in the treatment of menorrhagia. J Am Assoc Gynecol Laparosc 2002;9(4):418-28

Gallinat A, Nugent W. NovaSure™ Impedance-controlled system for endometrial ablation. J Am Assoc Gynecol Laparosc 2002;9(3):279-85

Busund B, Erno LE, Gronmark A, Istre O. Endometrial ablation with NovaSure™ GEA, a pilot study. Acta Obstet Gynecol Scand 2003;82(1):65-8

Fulop T, Rakoczi I, Barna I. NovaSure™ Impedance Controlled Endometrial Ablation System. Long-Term Follow-up Results. Proceedings of the Second World Congress on Controversies in Obstetrics, Gynecology & Infertility Vol. II, Paris, France 2001;pp149-155

Laberge PY, Sabbah R, Fortin C, Gallinat A. Assessment and comparison of intra- and postoperative pain associated with NovaSure™ and ThermaChoice endometrial ablation systems. J Am Assoc Gynecol Laparosc 2003;10(2):223-32

Cooper J, Skalnyi E. Radiofrequency endometrial ablation systems. In: Bieber E, Loffer F. editors. Hysteroscopy, Resectoscopy and Endometrial Ablation. The Parthenon Publishing Group. 2003;p.191-4

REPEAT ENDOMETRIAL ABLATION

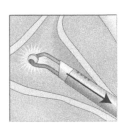

Richard J. Gimpelson, M.D., P.C.

Endometrial ablation is an excellent alternative to hysterectomy for women with prolonged or heavy uterine bleeding and in whom hormonal therapy is unsuccessful, undesired, or contraindicated. Endometrial ablation by many methods will be successful up to 90% of the time. Women in whom the procedure is not successful have the choice of hysterectomy, observation, or repeat ablation.

INDICATIONS

The indications for repeat endometrial ablation will be one of five categories:

1. Uterine bleeding improved, but still heavy or prolonged and adversely affecting the patient's quality of life;

2. Physical or mental disability in which amenorrhea is desired;

3. Initial procedure not completed because of excess fluid absorption, leiomyomas, instrument malfunction, or uterine perforation;

4. Amenorrhea desired by patient despite achieving reduced or normal flow;

5.   Unimproved.

Repeat ablation is usually indicated for those patients found in category 1, although all categories can be managed in a similar manner.

ANATOMY

Complete knowledge of uterine anatomy is essential prior to undertaking a repeat ablation. The uterine cavity will often be shaped quite differently in the ablated cavity, as compared to the unablated cavity. Following endometrial ablation (even unsuccessful ones) the uterine cavity assumes a more narrow and cylindrical shape (Figure 1). Cornua are usually obliterated and obscured by adhesions. The myometrium may be thinner and the endometrium is quite variable, ranging from thick to absent. The uterus will often sound to a shorter length.

WORKUP

Once the decision is made to undergo repeat ablation, a series of steps should be undertaken to enhance success and reduce the risk of complications. A thorough history must be taken to fully assess the nature of the patient's bleeding pattern and to explain to the patient that even with a repeat procedure, amenorrhea cannot be guaranteed, although it is usually achieved 65% to 70% of the time.

A physical exam must be done including a PAP smear. If one suspects

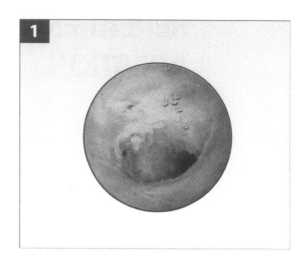

a bleeding disorder, appropriate tests should be ordered if not done with the first ablation.

A transvaginal ultrasound should be performed preferably by the gynecologist who will do the repeat ablation. This ultrasound is necessary to obtain valuable information on overall uterine size, to observe development of leiomyomas since initial procedure, and to look for hematometra or pockets of blood in the uterine cavity. In addition, the ultrasound will give the measurements of the overall uterine length, the uterine cavity length, the uterine position, and myometrial thickness. The ultrasound will also allow evaluation for adnexal disease that would change the patient's management.

A hysteroscopic exam and endometrial sampling must be done prior to the repeat ablation. If it has been less than one year since the initial ablation, the hysteroscopy, endometrial sampling, and repeat ablation can be performed at the same time. If it has been over one year, the evaluation should be done as a separate procedure from the repeat ablation. Repeat ablation is performed with either Nd:YAG laser or a roller electrode can be used if the cavity is large enough. One should wait at least six months after the first ablation to allow full healing of the uterus before considering a repeat ablation.

DIAGNOSTIC HYSTEROSCOPY

A 5.5 mm or smaller continuous flow hysteroscope should be used for the diagnostic workup if saline is used for distention media. An even smaller caliber sheath can be used if CO_2 distention is preferred. Insertion of the hysteroscope should first be attempted under direct vision before sounding or dilatation to reduce the risk of uterine perforation. The operator must be familiar with the uterine size and positioning as discovered on the transvaginal ultrasound results prior to the procedure. If the hysteroscope cannot be advanced into the uterine cavity, an alternate method must be carried out. A sound dilator (Cooper Surgical, Shelton, CT) (Figure 2) will allow one to enter the uterine cavity with minimal risk of perforation. This device is a narrow sound with a 2 mm tip and expanding to a 4 mm diameter with one centimeter marks and more prominent marks at five, ten, fifteen, and twenty centimeters. This instrument allows the operator to carefully create a cavity. If a perforation occurs, the chance of other

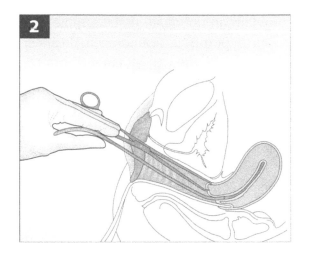

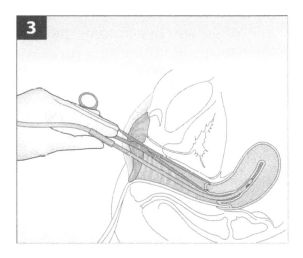

organ injury is minimal, but the procedure should be halted and the patient observed until stable.

Once a small passage is created with the hysteroscope, suction curettage can be performed. If the sound dilator is used to create a cavity, further careful dilation to a 5 mm diameter should be performed. Once dilation reaches 5 mm, the hysteroscope may be inserted into the uterine cavity. After viewing the uterine cavity, suction curettage (Milex Products, Chicago, IL) (Figure 3) will obtain an adequate tissue sample to rule out hyperplasia or endometrial cancer.

Do not use a sharp curette, as it is not as thorough as the suction curette at sampling the uterus or at removing excess tissue. When the pathology report is returned as benign, a repeat endometrial ablation may be scheduled.

REPEAT ABLATION TECHNIQUE

The initial entry into the uterine cavity is achieved in the same manner as the diagnostic hysteroscopy procedure described here. However, a paracervical block with 0.25 % Bupivacine should be administered to reduce post-operative discomfort, even if the procedure is performed under general anesthesia.

Preparation of the endometrium is performed mechanically by a suction curettage for 2 to 3 minutes. This will give a visual end point as the roughened red surface (Figure 4) will show a definite response to electrical or laser energy. There is no need for medical preparation of the endometrium prior to repeat ablation. Do not use any of the global ablation devices for repeat endometrial ablation because repeat ablation should be carried out under clear direct vision.

A 21 Fr or smaller operating hysteroscopy sheath can be used with the Nd:YAG laser. If the roller electrode is used, a larger sheath is needed.

Cervical and uterine cavity dilation will need to be carried out carefully.

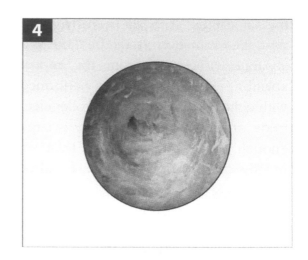

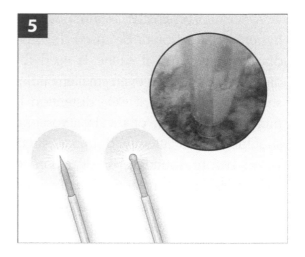

ND:YAG LASER

The Nd:YAG laser is the ideal instrument for repeat endometrial ablation. The bare fiber (either straight directed or 70° directed) can be used depending on the operator's preference. The laser should be applied in a non-touch technique when possible to create an obvious visual end point of white blanching (Figure 5). The power is set at 50 W and the laser is slowly moved to "paint" the entire uterine cavity down to the internal cervical os. Be careful to continuously, but slowly, move the fiber to avoid directing too much laser energy into one area and possibly cause cavitation of the myometrium. The uterine cavity after repeat ablation is shown on Figure 6.

ROLLER ELECTRODE

If the cavity is large enough, a roller electrode can be used for repeat endometrial ablation. The same mechanical preparation is carried out as for the Nd:YAG laser. Medical preparation may be used (Lupron Depot 3.75 mg). However, this will often reduce the uterine cavity size and cervical canal to a point that entry may be difficult. Power should be at 70 W cutting and 70 W coagulation and the same technique as for initial ablation should be used. The roller should always be drawn toward the lower uterine segment and never advanced toward the fundus while energy is delivered (Figure 7).

Once the procedure is completed, the patient will be observed for one to two hours and then discharged. Patients are given Toradol 30 mg IV before or during the procedure and discharged on non-steroidal anti-inflammatory drugs and or narcotics if needed. All patients are given diphenhydramine HCl 50 mg immediately post-op and then again at 6 hours and 12 hours post-procedure. The addition of diphenhydramine HCl has markedly reduced the patient's post-operative discomfort,

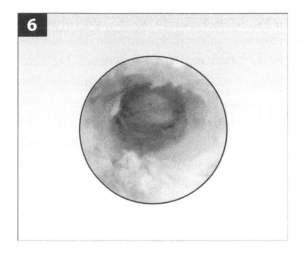

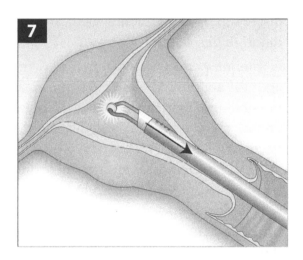

probably due to its multiple effects of sedation, augmentation of pain relief, anti-inflammation and anti-nausea. In addition, diphenhydramine HCl has a very high margin of safety.

COMPLICATIONS

Repeat endometrial ablation has the same potential complications as the initial procedure: fluid overload, perforation, bleeding, infection, and thermal injury to structures outside the uterus. Fluid overload can be avoided by carefully monitoring the inflow and outflow of distention media. Utilization of one of the fluid monitoring devices commercially available minimizes this risk. Electrolytes should be measured before the procedure for comparison if excess fluid absorption is suspected during the procedure. Bleeding and infection are very unlikely to occur and prophylactic antibiotics can be given at the operator's discretion as the patient's medical condition might warrant.

Uterine perforation and thermal damage to abdominal structures are real possibilities. Extreme care in the initial uterine entry, sounding, and dilatation is necessary. Referral back to the pre-operative ultrasound is a must to note the uterine size, cavity length, and uterine positioning. Perforation will still occur on occasion with repeat ablations, and the procedure must be stopped at that point. If laser or electrical energy is being used at the time of the perforation, assessment for abdominal injury must be proceeded by laparoscopy or laparotomy. If perforation occurs from sounding, dilatation, or insertion of the hysteroscope, then the procedure must be terminated and the patient brought back in three months for another repeat procedure, or another method may be needed to treat the bleeding.

There is very little discomfort one day after repeat ablation. If one is notified by the patient of complaints other than mild cramping (e.g., severe pain, nausea, vomiting, bloating), the patient should be seen and evaluated for possible endometritis or abdominal injury.

WARNING

Repeat endometrial ablation is not as easy a procedure as the initial ablation, and if one gynecologist in a region is adept at repeat ablation, it is often best to refer patients to that gynecologist.

SUGGESTED READING:

Loffer FD. Hysteroscopic endometrial ablation with the Nd:YAG laser using a non-touch technique. Obstet Gynecol 1987;69:679-682

Gimpelson RJ, Kaigh J. Endometrial ablation: repeat procedures. J Reprod Med1992;37:629-635

Gimpelson RJ, Kaigh J. Mechanical preparation of the endometrium prior to endometrial ablation. J Reprod Med 1992;37 691-694

Gimpelson RJ. Role of Second-look Resectoscope and Repeat Procedures. In: Bieber EJ, Loffer FD (eds) Gynecologic Resectoscopy, Cambridge: Blackwell Science, 1995:254-268

HYSTEROSCOPIC SURGERY: INDICATIONS, CONTRAINDICATIONS AND COMPLICATIONS

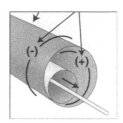

George A. Vilos, M.D.

INDICATIONS FOR HYSTEROSCOPY/SURGERY

There are several indications for hysteroscopy:

Direct visualization of the endometrial cavity for assessment and sampling, when indicated, in women with menstrual or fertility disorders.

Diagnostic hysteroscopy and biopsy in women with abnormal uterine bleeding is indicated when one is unable to perform an office biopsy or the sample is inadequate or inconclusive.

Direct surgical access for intrauterine surgery versus trans-abdominal and/or trans-uterine surgery for removal of foreign body (misplaced intrauterine contraceptive devices) and for therapy of endometrial polyps, intracavitary, submucosal and some intramural fibroids, division of intrauterine adhesions and septa, tubal cannulation for proximal tubal disease, tubal occlusion for family planning and finally treatment of abnormal uterine bleeding by ablating or resecting the endometrium.

CONTRAINDICATIONS TO HYSTEROSCOPY/SURGERY

- Limited knowledge of the instruments and equipment required for surgery;

- The proposed surgery is beyond the surgeon's experience and expertise;

- The patient is not a suitable surgical candidate;

- Medical conditions precluding hysteroscopic surgery and the use of associated distention media and energy sources. For example, patients with renal disease may not tolerate any fluid absorption while cardiac pacemakers may malfunction in the presence of high frequency (radiofrequency, RF) electrosurgery;

- Other uterine and/or pelvic pathology requiring additional surgical procedures such as hysterectomy and pelvic floor repairs;

- Lack of appropriate instrumentation and equipment;

- Unwillingness to consent after the risks and benefits have been explained;

- Acute pelvic inflammatory disease;

- Known genital tract malignancies;

- Known pregnancy;

- Inability to dilate the cervix;

- Inability to distend the uterus and obtain clear view.

INFORMED CONSENT

In the issue of informed consent the following should be discussed:

The nature, benefits and objectives of the proposed surgery;

Alternative therapeutic options including the consequences of no treatment;

The material risks and possible complications. A material risk is defined as a risk of high frequency (usually > 1%) or a risk that, although remote, may result in possible grave consequences such as death or major impairment;

Possible intra-operative findings and their management;

Complications associated with any kind of gynecological surgery such as anesthesia issues and surgical complications including infection, bleeding and injury to adjacent organs such as the genital tract, bladder, ureters, bowel and vessels;

The need for possible laparoscopy, laparotomy and even hysterectomy since some of these complications, such as perforations, excessive uncontrollable bleeding and thermal injury might require additional corrective surgery;

Realistic post-operative expectations;

Long-term implications of endometrial ablation and hormone replacement therapy;

Implications regarding fertility, family planning, inadvertent pregnancy and pregnancy outcomes following endometrial ablation;

Risk of requiring further medical or surgical therapy;

Complications specific to hysteroscopic surgery can be classified under:

Traumatic injuries;

Distending media complications;

Thermal injuries.

TRAUMATIC COMPLICATIONS

Cervical tears of varying degrees occur frequently during dilatation of the cervix. Such tears may lead to uncontrollable bleeding and if they extend into the broad ligament, bleeding may be significant and may warrant laparoscopy, laparotomy and possible hysterectomy.

False passages have been created by the dilator and/or the resectoscope into the uterine wall without complete perforation of the uterus. These false passages, if unrecognized, may lead to excessive bleeding, air embolism, fluid absorption and even injury to adjacent organs such as ureters and bladder.

Uterine perforation occurs at a frequency of 0.8% to 2%. In one study of 1952 women undergoing 2116 hysteroscopies there were 34 (1.61%) uterine perforations while in four published series involving 3154 hysteroscopic endometrial ablations there were 36 (1.14%) perforations. The American Association of Gynecologic Laparoscopists' 1993 membership survey involving 14,707 operative hysteroscopies reported a perforation rate of 1.42%. The uterine perforation rate increases up to 7% during repeat endometrial ablation. Uterine perforation with a dilator and/or the resectoscope may lead to excessive fluid absorption, bleeding and/or infection. The most significant part of this complication may be the inability to perform or complete the intended surgical procedure.

TIPS TO AVOID TRAUMATIC COMPLICATIONS

• When cervical stenosis is known or suspected such as in nulliparous patients, no previous vaginal delivery, postmenopausal women or pre-operative use of gonadotrophin releasing hormone agonists (GnRH-a) to thin the endometrium the surgeon might consider the insertion of a cervical laminaria tent at least four hours prior to surgery or vaginal misoprostol (200–400 mcg) 2–4 hours prior to surgery. The use of oral misoprostol is associated with systemic side effects and its use is controversial;

• Intra-operative pelvic examination is mandatory to determine the size, shape, mobility and especially the position of the uterus. The insertion of the uterine sound or the initial dilators should slide through the cervical canal without undue force;

• The use of intra-cervical injection of a local anesthetic with dilute vasopressin or epinephrine (e.g., 10 mL, 0.5% Xylocaine with 1 in 200,000 epinephrine) appears to soften the cervix and facilitate dilatation;

• Consider the use of half size dilators and apply gentle steady force as the size of the dilators increases;

• When resistance is encountered, especially with the initial dilator, do not force the dilator. Direct visualization of the cervical canal with a small diameter hysteroscope usually identifies the opening of the cervical canal and the initial dilator(s) may be advanced under direct visualization.

TIPS PRIOR TO THE CONDUCT OF SURGERY:

• The patient should be provided with adequate analgesia/anesthesia. When local paracervical block is used it is imperative that one waits for several minutes for the local injection to take effect.

• The surgeon should assemble and inspect all the instruments to be used in the procedure.

• The surgeon should be familiar with all the equipment, their function, their required settings and their limitations including the distending media and the energy source used.

• The patient should be appropriately prepped and draped in the horizontal position on the operating table.

• The surgeon should perform a pelvic examination.

• The surgeon should sound the uterus and dilate the cervix.

• Observe the insertion of the hysteroscope on the TV monitor following the direction of the cervical canal.

• Ensure adequate distention/irrigant media for optimum/clear visualization;

• Ensure that only the endometrial cavity has been accessed by identifying the two tubal ostia, the internal cervical os and the cervical canal.

DISTENDING MEDIA COMPLICATIONS

AIR/CO_2/GAS EMBOLISM

Mechanical trauma to the cervix, creation of false passages, uterine perforations and breaching the integrity of subendometrial uterine vessels by coagulation or resection may allow the intravasation of room air, CO_2 distention media and/or gas bubbles generated at the time of surgery. The true incidence of air and/or gas embolism is unknown and is probably underestimated. Minor, nonlethal, cases may not be reported and other cases may be misdiagnosed as pulmonary emboli. Air embolism occurs when a non-collapsible vein is opened or severed and a positive pressure gradient is built up between the vessel and the ambient pressure or a negative pressure is generated between an open vessel and the heart. Gas emboli are usually filtered by the pulmonary capillary bed, leaving the patient asymptomatic. In pigs, air infused directly into the right ventricle at the rate of 0.05 mL/kg/min was completely filtered.

When the patient is in the Trendelenburg position, gas bubbles may be trapped in the splanchnic circulation, liver or left ventricle for a long time and only later produce symptoms of air embolism.

SIGNS AND SYMPTOMS OF AIR EMBOLISM

THE ANESTHETIST MAY BE THE FIRST TO NOTE THE FOLLOWING SIGNS:

- SUDDEN FALL OF OXYGEN SATURATION;
- DECREASED END TIDAL CO_2 VOLUME;
- HYPOTENSION;
- TACHYCARDIA;
- "METALLIC HEART" SOUNDS AND/OR A "MILL-WHEEL" MURMUR ON AUSCULTATION;
- THE DIAGNOSIS MAY BE CONFIRMED BY ECHOCARDIOGRAM OR TRANSESOPHAGEAL OR DOPPLER ULTRASOUND.

STRATEGIES FOR THE MANAGEMENT OF AIR EMBOLISM

PREVENTION

Avoid Trendelenburg position. When the heart level is below the uterus a negative pressure gradient is created and air is sucked in by open intrauterine veins;

Leave the last dilator in the cervix until ready to insert the hysteroscope;

Purge all air from inflow tubing at start and when changing distention media bags;

Minimize repetitive insertions of the resectoscope;

Use outflow suction (80 to 100 mmHg) to evacuate generated bubbles;

Avoid the use of non-collapsible distention media containers such as glass or solid plastic bottles;

Avoid the use of gases as distention media for operative hysteroscopy.

THERAPY

Undertake measures to curtail gas accumulation by immediate procedure cessation, with consequent elimination of the gas source;

Ventilate with 100% oxygen and infuse IV fluids to counteract hemoconcentration. Avoid diuretics and vasodilators;

Turn patient on her left side;

Intravenous steroids are recommended but convincing evidence for their efficacy is lacking;

Insert central venous pressure (CVP) line and aspirate the air from the right ventricle;

Use hyperbaric chamber for hyperbaric oxygenation if available (Boyle's law of gases, Pressure x Volume = constant).

DISTENDING FLUID MEDIA ISSUES

Uterine distention and irrigation is usually achieved by the use of normal saline when laser fiber systems or bipolar electrosurgery is used. Electrolyte-free solutions, such as sugars or amino acids, are required for the use of monopolar high frequency electrosurgical generators. Excessive, rapid and unpredictable absorption of such solutions leading to electrolyte changes, pulmonary and brain edema which may result in coma and even death, is one of the most serious complications of hysteroscopic surgery.

To prevent or minimize the risk of occurrence and to anticipate, recognize and effectively treat such complications the surgeon should be familiar with several principles including the physiology, physical and chemical properties, and the biochemistry and metabolism of the fluid used. Based on such basic knowledge the signs and symptoms exhibited during or following excessive fluid absorption can be anticipated and readily treated accordingly. Therefore, the surgeon should be familiar with strategies to institute effective therapies should such complications occur.

NORMAL FLUID PHYSIOLOGY

Fluid movement through tissue and into the vascular compartment follows the well-known principle of physiology hypothesized by E. H. Starling at the beginning of the last century. Starling proposed that under normal conditions a state of near equilibrium exists at the capillary arteriovenous network whereby the amount of fluid filtering outwards through the arterial capillaries equals the amount of fluid reabsorbed by the venous capillaries.

THE FIVE MAJOR FACTORS THAT REGULATE TRANSCAPILLARY MOVEMENT OF FLUID ARE:

• The mean capillary hydrostatic pressure (range 15–25 mmHg). This is directly proportional to the mean arterial pressure (MAP) of the patient and tends to push fluid out of the vessels;

• The interstitial fluid pressure (turgor pressure, range 5–7 mmHg), which tends to move fluid into the vessel;

• The capillary plasma colloid osmotic pressure (range 24–32 mmHg), which tends to cause osmosis of fluid into the vessel;

• The interstitial fluid colloid osmotic pressure (range 4–6 mmHg), which tends to cause osmosis of fluid out of the vessel;

• The permeability of the capillary membranes which varies greatly from one tissue to another.

During hysteroscopic surgery additional factors may alter the Starling equilibrium and/or contribute to excessive intravasation of fluid. The following factors have correlated with excessive fluid absorption:

• The intrauterine distention pressure (> MAP);

• The depth of tissue destruction or exposure of venous channels by direct transection, causing rapid intravasation. Endometrial resection allows more absorption than rollerball ablation;

- Increased intrauterine surface area related to uterine size. Uterine cavity depth > 12 cm;
- The duration of the surgical procedure;
- The tissue vascularity as seen in the presence of multiple submucous myomas;
- The temperature of the distention media;
- The volume of irrigant solution used;

The net fluid filtration coefficient from the uterine cavity into the vascular compartment is expressed in mL of fluid/min/mmHg/100 gm of tissue.

FACTORS AFFECTING FLUID INTRAVASATION AND THEIR EFFECTS

PRETREATMENT WITH GNRH ANALOGUE

A large randomized, double-blind study, comparing goserelin acetate (3.8 mg at 6 and 2 weeks pre-endometrial resection) versus placebo demonstrated 33% reduction in fluid absorption in the GnRH-a treated women (median fluid absorption 150 mL versus 225 mL, respectively);

INTRACERVICAL VASOPRESSORS

In at least three randomized, placebo controlled trials the administration of dilute pitressin solution (0.05–0.4 U/mL, total 20 mL) into the cervical stroma sig-nificantly reduced distention fluid intravasation by approximately 50%. The optimum effective dose of vaso-pressin for gynecologic surgery should not exceed 0.4 U/mL and the total pressor units should not exceed 4. The use of pitressin should be individualized and it should not be used indiscriminately. In animals, vasopressin increas-es total peripheral resistance and pul-monary vascular resistance and decreas-es cardiac output and coronary blood flow by 35–50%. Indeed, intra-operative myocardial infarction has been reported within minutes of a paracervical injec-tion of 5 mL of dilute vasopressin (4.29 U/mL). Furthermore, during an attempt-ed laparoscopic myomectomy a woman developed acute hypotension from coronary artery spasm and ventricular dyskinesia following a third injection of 3–5 mL of dilute vasopressin (0.6 U/mL). The use of vasopressin to reduce the risk of fluid intravasation has also been severely criticized because of its antidi-uretic effect and water retention.

INTRAUTERINE PRESSURE

The Starling equilibrium is adversely disturbed by any intrauterine pressure, with greater intrauterine pressure caus-ing greater fluid absorption. Therefore, one should use the lowest intrauterine pressure necessary to provide adequate visualization. It has been demonstrated that fluid absorption increases signifi-cantly when intrauterine pressure exceeds the mean arterial pressure (MAP) of the patient.

The median threshold pressure at which fluid spills through the fallopian tubes is approximately 100 mmHg and no spill occurs at pressures less than 70 mmHg. This indicates that an effective intrauterine pressure to distend the uterine cavity should be between 40 and 80 mmHg which is below the mean arterial pressure of the patient (MAP normally > than 80 mmHg). As the intrauterine pressure increases higher fluid absorption occurs at an approximate rate of 1.5 mL/mmHg.

When a gravity delivery system is used the bag should be placed approximately 1 m (100 cm H_2O, equivalent to 75 mmHg pressure) above the patient's pelvis and connected to a suction outflow of approximately 100-mmHg negative pressure (Figure 1). Commercially available infusion pumps regulate the media infusion rate as well as the inflow and outflow pressures while continuously monitoring fluid deficit.

OUTFLOW SUCTION

The use of suction to the outflow of irrigant solution markedly reduces intravasation of irrigant fluid and maintains a clearer view by evacuating generated bubbles and surgical debris.

COMMONLY USED FLUIDS

The two basic physiological princi-

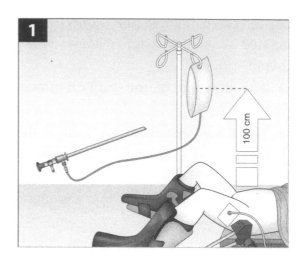

ples governing the regulation of body fluids are: 1) osmotic equilibrium and 2) ionic strength. Therefore, the surgeon should select the most appropriate irrigant solution which is least likely to cause serious complications should it be absorbed. Ideally, the irrigant fluid should be isonatremic and isotonic such as normal saline or Ringer's lactate. However, the use of normal saline with bipolar electrosurgical and laser fiber systems does not preclude excessive absorption of fluid and should not lull one into a false sense of security. Saline is absorbed at the same rate, and under the same conditions as other fluids, and at least one death has occurred from pulmonary and brain edema following excessive absorption of normal saline during hysteroscopic myomectomy.

Unipolar electrosurgery requires the use of non-conducting (non-electrolytic) solutions. Amino acid or sugar solutions alone, or in combination, are commonly used solutions that are non-conducting. Regardless of the solution used, the surgeon should know its physiology, physical properties and biochemistry and metabolism.

GLYCINE

Glycine (1.5%, 3%), a nonessential amino acid, is a distention/irrigant solution used frequently by both urologists and gynecologists. It is an acidic and hypotonic solution. It is rapidly metabolized directly by oxidative deamination into a ketoacid (CH_3COOH) and ammonia (NH_3+) or via intermediate aminoacids such as serine which by itself may cause encephalopathy if found in excess concentrations. Ammonia is normally excreted through the urea cycle but under certain conditions it can similarly cause encephalopathy. The ketoacid CH_3COOH further metabolizes into carbon dioxide (CO_2) and free water (H_2O). The CO_2 forms carbonic acid while the free water causes dilutional hyponatremia. Therefore, excessive absorption of glycine results in acidemia, hypo-osmolality, electrolyte changes (hyponatremia) and hyperammonemia (Figure 2). These changes may cause cardiac arrhythmias as well as pulmonary and brain edema which may result in blindness, brain stem herniation and ultimately death.

SORBITOL

Sorbitol 3.3% is a hypotonic (165 mOsm/L) sugar solution. If absorbed in excess it causes hyperglycemia. It is

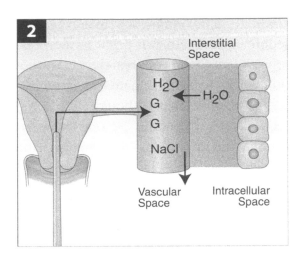

metabolized into carbon dioxide and water resulting in acidemia and dilutional hyponatremia.

MANNITOL

Mannitol is a six-carbon alditol isomer solution. It is isotonic (275 mOsm/L) and electrolyte-free. Once absorbed, less than 10% is metabolized with the remainder filtered by the kidneys and excreted in urine by osmotic diuresis. The plasma half-life is 15 to 20 minutes. Excessive intravasation results in dilutional hyponatremia but because it is isoosmotic and also causes its own diuresis its use is advocated for preventing complications associated with acute hyponatremia, such as cerebral edema and brain stem herniation. However, it is unclear whether isotonic hyponatremia created by 5% mannitol is safer than hypotonic hyponatremia created by 1.5% glycine or 3% sorbitol. The exact control of fluid and electrolyte movement across brain cells is very complex.

Chapter 20

246 | HYSTEROSCOPIC SURGERY: INDICATIONS, CONTRAINDICATIONS AND COMPLICATIONS ....

Animal data suggests that cerebral edema and death can occur in the presence of isotonic hyponatremia. A study involving acute hyponatremia in rabbits demonstrated that although less brain edema occurred with isotonic hyponatremia the mortality rate remained the same, approximately 30%.

SIGNS AND SYMPTOMS OF ACUTE HYPONATREMIA

The signs and symptoms of hyponatremia include nausea, vomiting, headache and disorientation. Patients may become obtunded, and may progress into muscle twitching, seizures, coma, respiratory arrest and death due to herniation of the brain stem.

In addition to hyponatremia and hyperammonemia serum biochemical changes may include transient hyperglycinemia (and some other amino acids), blood oxygen desaturation, hypercapnia, coagulopathy and mild hemolysis.

The normal mean concentration of serum sodium is 140 mmol/L (range 135–145). Hyponatremia is defined as serum Na+ < 130 mmol/L. When serum Na+ falls below 120 mmol/L hyponatremia is considered severe and corrective measures should be considered. Patients with serum Na+ < 100 mmol/L are at grave risk of brain impairment and/or death. One study in men undergoing transurethral prostatectomy (TURP) estimated that absorption of 1 L of 1.5% glycine was associated with a decrease of serum Na+ of 4 to 8 mmol/L. Studies in women have shown that serum Na+ falls approximately 10 mEq/L for every 1000 mL of glycine absorbed and hyponatremia correlated to glycine deficit.

It has been estimated that premenopausal women are 25 times more likely to sustain permanent brain damage or die from hyponatremic encephalopathy than are postmenopausal women or men. The mortality rate in these women was 21%. These observations imply that the presence of estrogen has a significant and deleterious effect. Indeed, animal studies suggest that the ionic pump responsible for homeostasis of brain cells is adversely affected by sex hormones accounting for the increased morbidity of hyponatremia in premenopausal women. Changes in the ionic pump may be compounded or a similar one caused by elevated post-operative levels of vasopressin. In rats it has also been shown that estrogen causes release of vasopressin, whereas testosterone inhibits it. Increased levels of vasopressin results in enhanced water retention with retarded Na+, K+-ATPase activity.

Furthermore, in a randomized, placebo controlled study, the Na+, K+-ATPase pump activity was significantly increased in GnRH-a treated patients compared to saline controls. The correlation between this increase and the decrease in estradiol levels was significant. Vasopressin levels were also significantly suppressed in the GnRH-a group compared to the placebo group and remained suppressed in the GnRH-a group, whereas the placebo group had increased levels post-operatively. The decrease correlated with endogenous serum estradiol levels.

Other studies have demonstrated that the Na+, K+-ATPase pump in specific regions of the brain is sensitive to estrogen and progesterone and animal studies show that the pump is less effective in females and leads to deregulation of cerebral fluid and electrolyte homeostasis. The Na+, K+-ATPase activity in rat brain varies significantly during the reproductive cycle and decreases with estrogen treatment. Gonadal steroids affect this activity in myocardium, kidneys, ileum and liver which may contribute to the pathophysiology of fluid overload and death and may explain the increased susceptibility of women to hyponatremia.

STRATEGIES TO MINIMIZE THE ESTROGEN EFFECTS

These observations allow the development of strategies not only to minimize excessive fluid absorption but to reduce the clinical effects of inadvertently absorbed fluids. These strategies include:

• Perform hysteroscopic surgery in the immediate postmenstrual period when serum estrogen levels and endometrial thickness are at their minimum.

• Surgery may be scheduled approximately 28 days after one package of oral contraceptives;

• Pre-treat patients with danazol 100–600 mg daily 2 to 4 months prior to surgery;

• Pre-treat patients with a GnRH-a 1 to 3 months prior to surgery.

In one randomized, placebo controlled study, goserelin acetate (3.6 mg) at 6 and 2 weeks prior to hysteroscopic endometrial ablation/resection thinned the endometrium (1.6 mm v 3.4 mm), reduced surgery time by 22%, reduced fluid absorption by 33% and increased amenorrhea rate (40% versus 26%).

GnRH-a also increases endometrial Na+, K+-ATPase pump activity possibly inhibiting estrogen mediated inactivity, thus creating an environment that is protective against hyponatremic encephalopathy.

Finally, GnRH-a suppresses the stress related release of vasopressin during or after surgery which may prevent further fluid absorption and hyponatremic complications

STRATEGIES TO TREAT HYPONATREMIA

It is recommended that chronic hyponatremia should not be corrected at a rate faster than 0.5 mEq/L/hour in order to avoid osmotic demyelination known as central pontine myelinolysis which is associated with devastating neurologic sequelae and high mortality.

However, acute hyponatremia associated with brain swelling, seizures and coma is life threatening and usually requires correction. Patients at risk of becoming symptomatic are those with serum Na+ < 120 mEq/L.

According to one study, the risk of developing hyponatremic encephalopathy did not depend on the absolute level of serum sodium, nor in the rapidity of the development of hyponatremia. The majority of patients who developed hyponatremic encephalopathy did so more than 24 hours post-operatively with serum Na+ values ranging from 116–128 mEq/L, implying additional factors involved in the development of this condition. Alternatively, the immediate cause of morbidity and death may be more a function of hypoosmolality than hyponatremia

TREATMENT OF SYMPTOMATIC PATIENTS

1. INTRAVENOUS INFUSION OF 1 L OF 0.9% SALINE OR RINGER'S LACTATE;

2. AGGRESSIVE DIURESIS WITH 20 TO 40 MG OF FUROSEMIDE OR MANNITOL;

3. SUPPLEMENTAL OXYGEN AND VENTILATORY SUPPORT IF THERE IS EVIDENCE OF PULMONARY CONGESTION/EDEMA;

4. MONITOR VITAL SIGNS, URINE OUTPUT, SERUM OSMOLALITY AND ELECTROLYTES, INCLUDING CALCIUM;

5. CONSIDER INFUSION OF SODIUM BICARBONATE (1–2 AMPULE(S)). ONE AMPULE CONTAINS 50 MEQ OF Na^+/50 mL OF SOLUTION.

6. CONSIDER HYPERTONIC SALINE INFUSION. THE USE OF HYPERTONIC SALINE (3%, 5%) IS CONTROVERSIAL BECAUSE RAPID CORRECTION MAY LEAD TO CENTRAL PONTINE MYELINOLYSIS.

TREATMENT OF ASYMPTOMATIC PATIENTS

1. RESTRICT INTAKE OF FLUIDS;

2. MONITOR SERUM Na^+, K^+ AND Ca^{++}. ALL THREE ELECTROLYTES MAY HAVE TO BE REPLACED;

3. CONSIDER DIURESIS WITH FUROSEMIDE (10 TO 20 MG IV) OR MANNITOL 0.5 MG/KG;

4. MONITOR INPUT AND OUTPUT OF FLUIDS

ONE WAY TO CALCULATE SALINE NEEDED

1. EXTRACELLULAR FLUID (ECF) $\approx$ 1/3 OF BODY WEIGHT (KG);

2. Na^+ DEFICIT $\approx$ (PRE-OP Na^+ - POST-OP Na^+) x ECF;

3. SALINE NEEDED $\approx$ $\dfrac{Na^+ \text{ DEFICIT (mEq/L)}}{514 \text{ (FOR 3\%) OR 855 mEq/L}}$ (FOR 5% SALINE)

4. E.G. 60 KG WOMAN, POST OP Na^+ = 100, Na^+ DEFICIT 40 mEq/L;

5. SALINE NEEDED
   ~ 800 + 5:14 ~ 1.5 L OF 3% SALINE
   ~ 800) 855 ~ 0.9 L OF 5% SALINE

6. RATE OF CORRECTION ~
   1 mEq/L/HOUR

7. DO NOT RAISE SERUM
   Na^+ > 130 MMOL/L

TIPS TO MINIMIZE EXCESSIVE FLUID ABSORPTION AND ITS SEQUELAE

• GnRH-a pretreatment reduces fluid absorption and the impact of absorbed fluids;

• Pharmacological thinning of the endometrium with oral contraceptives/danazol;

• Plan surgery in the immediate post-menstrual period;

• Intracervical injection of pressor agents (vasopressin, epinephrine);

• Use a distending pressure less than the patient's mean arterial pressure;

• Diligent monitoring of fluid deficit every 1000 mL of irrigant fluid used. (Do not go by time i.e. every 5 or 10 minutes. Absorption can occur very rapidly when large vessels are transected). Also bear in mind that all commercially available 3 L bag solutions contain 5% to 10% more than 3L;

• Establish a maximum allowable fluid absorption (MAFA) for each patient prior to the procedure and ensure that the threshold is not exceeded. Allow approximately 20 mL/kg including the fluid infused intravenously.

RESPONSE TO NON-ELECTROLYTIC FLUID DEFICIT

• DEFICIT ~ 1000 mL. COMPLETE PROCEDURE EXPEDITIOUSLY AND EVALUATE ELECTROLYTES;

• DEFICIT > 1500 mL Na^+ < 125 mEq/L

• TERMINATE PROCEDURE, EVALUATE ELECTROLYTES AND CONSIDER DIURESIS;

• THE CORRESPONDING VOLUMES IF NORMAL SALINE IS USED ARE 2000 AND 2500 mL, RESPECTIVELY.

THERMAL INJURIES

HOT WEIGHTED SPECULUM BURNS

Ovoid buttock burns, approximately 2 x 4 cm area, have been encountered in three obese women (> 200 lb) undergoing ThermaChoice balloon ablation, resectoscopic rollerball ablation and vaginal hysterectomy. Experiments demonstrated that the weighted speculum cools off differentially with the ball temperature remaining > 45° in room air for at least 30 minutes after autoclaving. The speculum cools to < 40° within one minute when rinsed or bathed with at least 1 L of saline solution.

THE BASICS OF ELECTROSURGERY

ELECTROSURGICAL UNIT (ESU)

All modern electrosurgical generators have safety features including isolated circuitry, balanced output of power, and return electrode monitoring (REM) system. They are not Bovie generators. William Bovie (a physicist) took the household electrical current (frequency 60 Hz) and transformed the frequency up to 300,000–500,000 Hz. This high frequency-called radio frequency (RF)-does not electrocute the patient nor stimulate muscles and/or nerves. The Bovie generator was ground referenced. This means the circuit was completed from the generator to the active electrode, to the patient's tissue, and from the patient to the ground through the ground plate attached to the patient's buttocks or thighs (Figure 3). All modern generators are isolated. i.e. they are not ground referenced. The circuit is completed from the generator to the active electrode (pencil or instrument), to the patient, and back to the generator through the dispersive pad electrode attached to the thigh or buttocks (Figure 4).

RETURN ELECTRODE MONITORING (REM) SYSTEM

Return dispersive electrode pads range from 90 to 126 cm^2, surface area, which is large enough to prevent dangerous concentrations at the point

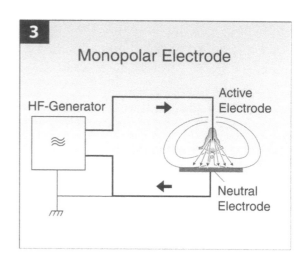

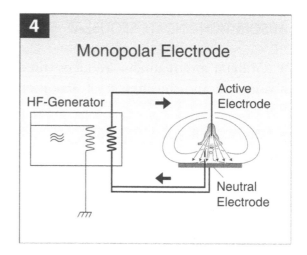

where the current exits the patient to return to the generator. Complications can occur. For instance, the electrode can become partially detached due to adhesive failure. If the electrode contact isn't completely touching the skin because of excessive hair, a bony prominence, or other causes, the contact impedance increases and more electricity is forced through the area of the pad still in contact with the patient. The increased current concentration through the smaller contact area will generate localized heat, resulting in a severe burn.

The heat factor (HF) equals the current squared x the time factor: $(HF=I^2 x\ t)$.

POWER, VOLTAGE, CURRENT, RESISTANCE (IMPEDANCE), POWER DENSITY, CAPACITANCE

Electrical current consists of a parade (flow) of electrons jumping along the ionized atoms or molecules of a conducting medium (solid, fluid or biological tissue) pushed by the force of voltage and opposed (resisted, impeded) by properties of the conductive medium. The flow of current (I) in Amperes (A) is directly proportional to the driving force (voltage) in volts (V) and inversely proportional to the resistance (R) offered by the conductor in ohms in accordance with Ohm's law: $I=V/R$.

Biologic tissues do not offer pure resistance such as that specific to various metal wires and other conductors since they have their own minimal electrical charge (measured in mV) and a component of capacitance as a result of cell membranes maintaining unequal distribution of ions across them. In addition, during electrosurgery tissue resistance constantly increases as tissue becomes heated and dehydrated (desiccated). Therefore, resistance offered by biologic tissue is referred to as impedance rather than resistance. Impedance measured in various biological tissues is

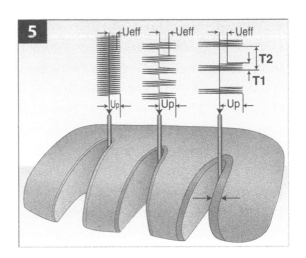

approximated to be 30 ohms for blood, 300 to 400 ohms for muscle, 1000 to 2000 ohms for fat, 1000 ohms for wet epithelium, and over 100,000 ohms for dry skin.

Two fundamental principles of electricity that apply to electrosurgery are of major importance: electrical current, given the opportunity, always flows to the return electrode or neutral plate (ground); and it follows the path of least resistance. These axioms and the concepts of current, current density, voltage, capacitance, power, capacitive coupling, and the way they affect tissue must be understood, together with necessary safety precautions.

A typical modern ESU is dialed or set by the operator (physician, nurse, etc) to deliver power waveforms in watts.

Power (W) = Voltage (V) x current (A)

Energy (J) = 1 W x 1 sec = 1 Joule

The ESUs are designed to deliver two waveforms of energy, a continuous waveform, low peak-to-peak voltage (<3500 V), used to cut; and an intermittent, modulated (damped) waveform (peak-to-peak) voltage up to 10,000 V (Figure 5). These intermittent bursts are delivered at 30,000 to 40,000 per second and are used to coagulate by desiccating tissue. By varying the time interval and peak-to-peak voltage of each burst of power one can create several combinations of waveforms called blended currents. Most ESUs deliver 5 modes: pure cut, blend 1, blend 2, blend 3, and coagulation waveforms. The corresponding delivery intervals/currents are 100%, 50%, 40%, 25% and 6% of the time. The ESU modes deliver the wattage displayed regardless of mode, and the number of joules is the same provided that the control settings are equal. Therefore, the pure cut mode will cut or vaporize tissue at a lower setting than blend or coagulation modes due to the continuous nature of the cut waveform.

Power density (PD) is power delivered in watts divided by the surface area of the active electrode-tissue interface. PD = W/cm^2

During hysteroscopic surgery the following electrosurgical injuries have been reported.

UTERINE PERFORATION AND INJURY TO INTRA-ABDOMINAL VISCERA

Injuries to bowel, bladder, large vessels and pelvic wall have been encountered by the rollerball and loop electrode;

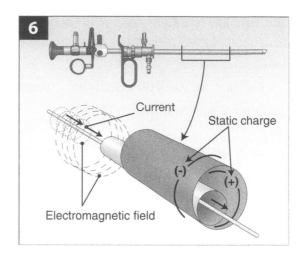

GENITAL TRACT INJURIES

Lower genital tract burns to cervix, vagina and vulva have been reported by unintended currents (unrecognized energy transfer or stray currents). Such currents may be generated by:

CAPACITIVE LEAKAGE CURRENT

The physics of the resectoscope arrangement unintentionally allows for a capacitor system. A capacitor is two nearby conductors separated by a non-conducting medium. The intended RF alternating current (AC) flowing through the active electrode and back to the ESU through the patient and the dispersive plate induces unintended (stray) RF current in the inner and outside sheaths of the resectoscope. This process is frequently referred to as the capacitance effect and it occurs without any direct electrical contact of the conductors (Figure 6).

INSULATION FAILURE (INSULATION BREAKS ALONG THE SHAFT OF THE ELECTRODES)

Resectoscopic electrodes (rollerballs, bars, loops etc) are insulated throughout their length except at the distal ball or loop and the proximal end attaching to the cable of the ESU. Insulation defects, not visually perceptible along the shaft of the electrode, can cause arcing (spark) or indirect coupling to the telescope thus electrifying the entire resectoscope.

We have measured the magnitude of the intended and stray currents of the resectoscope and their effects on biological tissue and have found that the potential for electrical/thermal burns to the genital tract during resectoscopic surgery is real. Capacitive coupled currents (20% to 25%) are induced onto the external sheath and may cause burns if the resectoscope/tissue interface area is small (< 3 cm^2), the power density is > 7.5 W/cm^2 and/or there is an over prolonged contact period. However, the most likely cause of the burns appears to be due to stray currents (arcing or direct contact) from defective electrode insulation to the telescope electrifying the entire resectoscope.

DISPERSIVE PAD INJURIES ASSOCIATED WITH HYSTEROSCOPIC SURGERY

During resectoscopic surgery dispersive pad burns to the thigh have been reported using REM dispersive pads and modern isolated generators.

One of the contributing factors was the inadvertent use of saline as an irrigant solution and excessive increase of the power output (watts) from a Valleylab Force 2 electrosurgical generator in accordance with HF=I^2 x t.

Other contributing factors may have been the progressive increase of current and prolonged activation of the generator in accordance with HF = I^2 x t.

CLINICAL TIPS TO MINIMIZE ELECTRICAL BURNS

• Inspect and ensure integrity of operating electrode and resectoscope. Electrodes are recommended for single use only;
• Use REM dispersive return electrodes;
• Never activate the electrode without appropriate visualization and proper orientation;
• Activate the electrode only when being withdrawn towards the cervix;
• Avoid prolonged activation intervals of the ESU and allow sufficient time between activation intervals to dissipate the heat built up at the dispersive electrode/skin interface (HF=I^2 x t);
• Avoid excessive power. Use the minimum effective power output to vaporize/cut the intended tissue (normally 80-120 W);
• Use two REM pads when higher power is required as with vaporizing myomas (cut power > 200 W);

• Electrical interference/diagonal lines on the TV monitor and/or patient twitching with electrode activation usually indicates electrical arcing. Stop and evaluate the electrical circuit;

• Do not increase the power setting if desired effect is not achieved. The following factors may be responsible:

  • incomplete/improperly connected circuit;

  • inadvertent use of a conducting solution such as saline or Ringer's lactate;

  • current diversion which may be burning the cervix, vagina or vulva;

• The smell of burning flesh is a late sign of genital tract burns;

• Consider the use of bipolar "technology" which requires a conducting solution and eliminates the need for return pad electrodes. This eliminates associated complications of monopolar electrosurgery, and the required non-conducting solutions;

• Create an in-service for nurses and physicians on the ESU use and limitations;

• Maintain in-house credentialing programs for basic electrosurgery;

• Establish protocols designed to minimize risks;

• Allow the ESU to cool down before using it for another procedure;

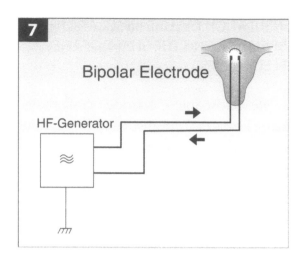

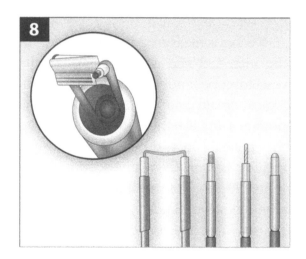

BIPOLAR TECHNOLOGY

The term "bipolar" technology has been introduced to describe the following: the surgeon grasps or touches the targeted tissue between two nearby conductors, usually 2–3 mm apart, where one performs as the active electrode and the other acts as the return electrode (Figure 7). All modern generators allow the use of both monopolar and bipolar modes individually or at the same time. The tissue in between is the only part of the patient included in the electrical circuit. Accordingly, a return (REM) electrode is no longer needed, and therefore there is no potential for a return electrode skin burn. Bipolar technology also eliminates the risk of current arcing, direct coupling, and capacitive coupling.

Unfortunately, bipolar electrosurgery works poorly with retracted blood vessels and thick tissue, and since the tissue to be coagulated must be placed between the active and return electrodes its use for hemostasis over a large surface area is limited. However, bipolar technology can be used under electrolytic solutions such as saline or Ringer's lactate.

In hysteroscopic surgery bipolar technology was first introduced as a small coaxial electrode (Versapoint™) using normal saline as irrigant solution. Presently, resectoscopes with larger vaporizing and cutting loop electrodes have been introduced (Figure 8). However, their safety remains to be demonstrated since no comparative studies with the traditional resectoscopes have been published.

CLINICAL SCENARIOS DURING HYSTEROSCOPIC SURGERY

EXCESSIVE BLOOD CLOTS, DEBRIS, ENDOMETRIUM:

Check for empty bag and inflow and outflow valves and tubes of the continuous irrigation system;

Wash out uterine cavity by inserting and withdrawing resectoscope;

Use the loop electrode (with no electricity) as a curette to remove, under direct vision clots, thick endometrium, tissue or resected tissue.

AIR OR GAS BUBBLES:

A large bubble in front of the telescope lens is air trapped under the insulating tip (beak) of the inner sheath of the resectoscope. Rotate the resectoscope 90° to 180° and the bubble will float upwards. Vigorous shaking of the resectoscope does not get rid of the air bubble.

Multiple gas bubbles obscure visibility at the fundus/anterior uterine wall. Remember the suction holes of the outside resectoscope sheath are at least one to two cm behind the telescope lens. To aspirate the bubbles advance the resectoscope past the bubbles rather than shaking the resectoscope vigorously.

INTRA-OPERATIVE LOSS OF VISIBILITY:

Check the entire irrigation/distention system (empty bag, inflow/outflow valves, etc); if distention/irrigation system is intact and the fluid is running assume uterine perforation until proven otherwise and act accordingly.

UTERINE PERFORATION

• If perforation with no electricity involved (uterine sound, dilator, resectoscope): expectant management (watch for excessive bleeding, consider antibiotics, etc); consider laparoscopic evaluation to assess for bleeding and remove excess fluid;

• If perforation with electricity involved or uncertain the pelvic organs should be assessed and the entire bowel should be examined via laparotomy or laparoscopy if able to do so.

RESECTION OF SUBMUCOUS MYOMAS

• Assess the size of the myoma by multiples of the 8 mm diameter loop;

Set power output at 100 W pure cut (continuous waveform);

Technique of resection; position loop, activate ESU and cut by pulling loop towards the cervix – never activate ESU and cut by pushing loop away from the cervix.

ACTIVATE GENERATOR AND THERE IS NO EFFECT ON TISSUE

• Check entire electrical circuit, all connections should be secure;

• Check distention/irrigation medium (saline/Ringer's may be the cause); do not increase power beyond recommended setting.

FLUID ABSORPTION

Example: Fifty minutes into the procedure, starting the 4th, 3 L bag of 1.5% glycine the anesthetist informs of ventilation problems and the nurse reports 1000 mL fluid deficit.

Steps:
• Stop procedure;
• Re-assess fluid deficit (bags > 3 L, 5–10% more);
• Draw blood for stat electrolytes; Infuse furosemide IV (20–40 mg);
• Foley catheter in bladder to monitor output.

BLEEDING COMPLICATIONS

PREVENTION:

• Pretreat patients with GnRH-a;
• Inject Vasopressors intracervically prior to surgery.

INTRA-OPERATIVE BLEEDING:

• Coagulate with rollerball or loop electrode;
• Bimanual compression of the uterus;
• Inject vasopressors intracervically.

POST-OPERATIVE BLEEDING:

IMMEDIATELY IN OPERATING ROOM (OR) (PATIENT STILL ANESTHETIZED);

• Bimanual compression of the uterus,
• Re-scope and coagulate with electrode,

- Inject vasopressor intracervically,

- Intrauterine Foley catheter and pressurize till bleeding stops (30–50 mL),

- Consider hysterectomy (vaginal or laparoscopic),

IN THE RECOVERY ROOM/SURGICAL DAYCARE FACILITY;

- Intrauterine Foley balloon and pressurize for at least 1 hour. After one hour desufflate Foley balloon: If no bleeding, remove Foley and discharge patient. If bleeding persists re-insufflate Foley and observe overnight. Consider antibiotic coverage,

- Back to OR for hysteroscopic coagulation or hysterectomy,

- Cyclokapron orally (500 mg bid x 4–5 days) (Tranexamic Acid – not available in the United States) similar in effect to Aminocaproic Acid as an antifibrinolytic,

- Transfemoral bilateral uterine artery occlusion.

DELAYED UTERINE BLEEDING (DAYS-WEEKS);

- Most likely due to infection (hemolytic streptococcus). Treat with antibiotics,

- Cyclokapron orally (500 mg bid x 4-5 days),

- Transfemoral uterine artery occlusion,

- Hysterectomy.

TO MINIMIZE THE RISK OF COMPLICATIONS DURING HYSTEROSCOPIC SURGERY PLEASE REMEMBER THE RULE OF 100'S ± 20

- SET THE INFLOW BAG AT 100 CM HEIGHT ABOVE PELVIS;

- SET THE OUTFLOW SUCTION AT 100 MMHG NEGATIVE PRESSURE;

- SET THE ESU POWER OUTPUT AT 100 W (CUT, BLEND OR COAG)

SUGGESTED READING:

Istre O, Skajaa K, Schjoensby A. Forman A. Changes in serum electrolytes after transcervical resection of endometrium and submucous fibroids with use of glycine 1.5% for uterine irrigation. Obstet Gynecol 1992;80:218-222

Istre O, Bjoennes J, Naess R, et al. Postoperative cerebral edema after transcervical endometrial resection and uterine irrigation with glycine. Lancet 1994;344:1187-1189

Ayus JC, Wheeler JM, Arieff AI. Postoperative hyponatremic encephalopathy in menstruant women. Ann Intern Med 1992;117:891-897

Taskin O, Buhur A, Birincioglu M, Burak F, Atmaca R, Yilmaz I, Wheeler JM. Endometrial Na+, k+ -ATPase pump function and vasopressin levels during hysteroscopic surgery in patients pretreated with GnRH agonists. J Am Assoc Gynecol Laparosc 1998;5:119-124

Fraser CL, Kucharcy ZKJ, Arieff AI, et al. Sex differences result in increased morbidity from hyponatremia in female rats. Am J Physiol 1989;256:R880-885

Arieff AI. Management of hyponatremia. Br Med J 1993;307:305-308

Vilos GA, Brown S, Grahan G, McCulloch S, Borg P. Genital tract electrical burns during hysteroscopic endometrial ablation: report of 13 cases in the United States and Canada. J Am Assoc Gynecol Laparosc 2000;7:141-47

Vilos GA, McCulloch S, Borg P, Zheng W, Denstedt J. Intended and stray radiofrequency electrical currents during resectoscopic surgery. J Am Assoc Gynecol Laparosc 2000;7:55-63

Raders JL, Vilos GA. Dispersive pad injuries associated with resectoscopic surgery. J Am Assoc Gyneco Laparosc 1999;6:363-367

Vilos GA. Intrauterine surgery using a new coaxial bipolar electrode in normal saline (Versapoint™): a pilot study. Fertil Steril 1999;72:740-743

INDEX

T - #0607 - 071024 - C0 - 254/190/13 - PB - 9780367394226 - Gloss Lamination